VARIATIONS IN GUIDED IMAGERY AND MUSIC:
TAKING A CLOSER LOOK

VARIATIONS IN GUIDED IMAGERY AND MUSIC:
TAKING A CLOSER LOOK

BRYAN MULLER

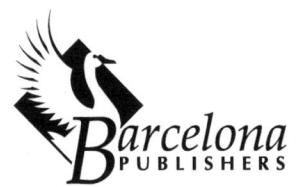

Variations in Guided Imagery and Music:
Taking a Closer Look

Copyright © 2014 by Barcelona Publishers

All rights reserved. No part of this book may be reproduced, reprinted, or distributed in any form whatsoever without written permission.

Print ISBN: 9781937440534
E-ISBN: 9781937440541

Distributed throughout the world by:
Barcelona Publishers
2427 Bond St.
University Park, IL 60484
866-620-6943
barcelonapublishers@gvtc.com
Website: www.barcelonapublishers.com
SAN 298-6299

Cover design:
© 2014 Frank McShane

Dedication

For Helen Bonny, whose love of music continues to resonate and inspire others to discover themselves. And, for those who are able to rediscover the Bonny Method again and again.

Acknowledgments

Thanks to Ken Bruscia for his dedication to Guided Imagery and Music and for teaching me to how to practice, research, and write about it.

Thanks to Cheryl Dileo for encouraging me to survey GIM fellows and for helping to make it a reality.

Table of Contents

Chapter One

The Creation Of Guided Imagery And Music/ 1
    Historical Perspectives/ 1
    Expansion and Development of the GIM Method/ 7

Chapter Two

The Main Components Of GIM And The Bonny Method/ 9
    State of Consciousness/ 11
    Spontaneous Imaging/ 12
    State of Consciousness and Spontaneous Imaging/ 13
    Classical Music Programs/ 14
    Goals/ 15
    Theoretical Orientation/ 17
    Verbal Dialogue/ 18
    Directive Interventions/ 18
    Length of Session and Music Experience/ 20
    Summary/ 21
    Table 1: Bonny's Individual Form and Modifications/ 22
    Table 2: Bonny's Group Form and Modifications/ 23

Chapter Three

Variations In Length Of Session And Music/ 25
    Most Frequent Practices/ 25
    Specific Practices/ 28
        Psychiatric/ 28
        Physical Illness/ 30
        Elderly/ 31
        Children and Adolescents/ 31
    Summary/ 32

Chapter Four

Variations In The Selection And Use Of Music/ 33
    Most Frequent Practices/ 33
    Specific Practices/ 34
        Psychiatric/ 35
        Physical Illness/ 38
        Elderly/ 39
        Children and Adolescents/ 39
        General-Purpose/ 40
    Summary/ 41

Chapter Five

Variations In Verbal Dialogue And Guiding/ 43
    Most Frequent Practices/ 43
    Specific Practices/ 45
        Psychiatric/ 45
        Physical Illness/ 49
        Elderly/ 62
        Children and Adolescents/ 52
        General-Purpose/ 54
    Summary/ 56

Chapter Six

Variations In Theoretical Orientation/ 57
    Most Frequent Practices/ 57
    Specific Practices/ 59
        Psychodynamic/ 59
        Jungian/ 63
    Summary/ 64

Table of Contents ix

Chapter Seven

GIM Combined With Other Techniques And Methods/ 65
    Specific Practices/ 65
        Neurolinguistic Programming / 66
        Gestalt Dreamwork/ 67
        Music, Drawing, and Narrative/ 68
        Spiritual Retreat/ 70
    Summary/ 71

Chapter Eight

Relationships Between Modifications/ 73
    Users of Bonny Method vs. Modifications/ 73
    Nondirective vs. Directive Interventions/ 74

Chapter Nine

Implications For Practice, Training, And Supervision/ 77
    Levels of Practice/ 77
        Supportive/ 78
        Intensive (Re-educative)/ 79
        Primary (Reconstructive)/ 80
    Modifications: Skill Levels/ 81
    Variations in Training and Supervision / 81
    Use of Terms/ 82

Chapter Ten

Summary/ 85
Length of Session and Music/ 85
Selection and Use of Music/ 85
Verbal Dialogue and Guiding/ 86

Theoretical Orientation/ 87
Bonny Method Practices and Modifications/ 87
On the Relationships between Variations/ 88
Implications/ 89
Closing Thoughts/ 90

References/ 93

Index/ 105

INTRODUCTION

Nearly four decades ago, Helen Bonny conceived of the use of music imaging in an altered state of consciousness while dialoguing with a trained guide for healing and self-actualization (Bonny & Goldberg, 2002). During 2009, from 317 to 557 individual and from 79 to 215 Group GIM sessions were offered each month worldwide, and it seems that these are very conservative estimates (Muller, 2010). Traditionally, *Guided Imagery and Music (GIM)* was used in private settings with adults and practiced within a humanistic orientation that emphasizes self-exploration and integration of all aspects of the self (Bonny, 2002g). Over time, practitioners explored more varied applications and uses of GIM. These new uses were shared amongst colleagues, discussed at conferences (Montgomery, 2012), and, with the advent of the Journal of the Association for Music and Imagery in 1992, more robustly presented in the literature. Over the past 30 years, uses of individual and Group GIM have been reported in a variety of settings, with children and adolescents, with the elderly, and with the physically and mentally ill (Bonny & Goldberg, 2002). In conjunction with this, modifications to Bonny's individual and group forms of GIM were reported. These included variations in the length of session and duration of music listening, variations in the selection and use of music, variations in verbal dialogue and guiding, the use of different theoretical orientations, and uses of the GIM method in combination with other therapeutic methods and techniques (Bonny & Goldberg, 2002; Bruscia, 2002a). By the end of the century, the breadth of GIM practices led to ambiguity, and there was a need to clarify the basic parameters of the method (Bruscia & Grocke, 2002). Bruscia's (2002a) chapter on boundaries—which is carefully based on Bonny's own writings—allowed modifications to be identified and distinguished from the Bonny Method of Guided Imagery and Music (BMGIM), and it allowed GIM practices to be distinguished from those belonging to music therapy and from those belonging to other professions. At that point, the incidence of the BMGIM and the modified practices it spawned was unknown. Based on distinctions provided by Bruscia (2002a), an anonymous electronic survey was designed to gather data regarding how frequently the original and modified forms of GIM were being utilized in practice (Muller, 2010). A key finding of this study was that Bruscia's boundaries are evident in the practices of GIM fellows.

The purpose of this book is to integrate the literature with the survey data and to consider some implications of the proliferation of modifications. This will be done in ten chapters. Chapter One, The Creation of Guided Imagery and Music, includes a synthesis of writings on Helen Bonny's life journey and how it led to the creation of GIM. Chapter Two, The Main

Components of GIM and the Bonny Method, includes a summary of Bruscia's (2002a) chapter on the Bonny Method and the boundaries of GIM. Chapters Three through Six include a review of the literature on modifications to the BMGIM paired with a summary of the frequency of their use in practice as revealed by the 2010 survey. Chapter Seven includes a review of the literature on the combined use of GIM with other methods and techniques. In Chapter Eight, Relationships between Modifications, the survey findings confirming the boundaries articulated by Bruscia (2002a), as well as those on the relationship between directive and nondirective interventions, are presented and discussed. Chapter Nine, Implications for Practice Training, and Supervision, includes a review of the literature on levels of practice, training, and supervision in GIM and a discussion about the use of terms. Finally, Chapter Ten includes a summary of the literature and data presented in chapters Three through Six, further discussion of implications, recommendations and closing thoughts. While reading these chapters, the reader is asked to approach them much like a GIM travel, to be open, and to consider all possibilities that efforts to extend the Bonny Method have raised.

It seems counterintuitive that a method which in its raw form contains so much flexibility has spawned so many modifications. Every phase of the BMGIM session (Prelude, Induction, Music Imaging, and Postlude) can already be adjusted in myriad ways to suit a client's needs. In fact, the BMGIM has been effective in treating clients with the same concerns (e.g., depression, PTSD) for whom modifications have been used (Meadows, 2002). That the BMGIM can be varied so much without losing its essential form is a testament to the wonder that led to its creation. That being said, sound clinical rationales have been presented for many modifications to Helen's method, but still, the proliferation of modifications raises some important questions: Has the potential of the BMGIM been fully understood or utilized? What defines mastery of the BMGIM? Is such mastery required for the practice of modifications? What is lost when the BMGIM is modified? To what extent are modifications informed by the BMGIM? As you consider these questions, and perhaps some others that come to mind as you read, ask yourself where you stand in relation to the BMGIM and modifications. Here are some positions to try: Modifications are needed because the BMGIM is inherently limited and modification is part of the natural evolution of the method. The BMGIM is fully evolved and understood, but it works only for certain clients, and modifications are necessary to accommodate their needs. We do not yet fully understand the potentials of the BMGIM or its applications, and thus we do not understand what may be lost through modification. These questions and positions are intended *not* to impose value judgments about the original method or any of its modifications, but to uncover them and to release their influence.

CHAPTER ONE

THE CREATION OF GUIDED IMAGERY AND MUSIC

Historical Perspectives

As Bonny (2002a) describes it, the experiences of her own life led her to the creation of Guided Imagery and Music (GIM). From infancy, her home life was filled with live music performed by her mother and later by herself and her siblings. From a young age, she was exposed to performances by the great classical artists of the time, and through her study of the violin, she became aware of what it meant to set intention and to live in the music. Disenchanted with the culture of teaching and performing classical music as a young adult, Bonny focused on raising a family. She continued to play the violin, and this, combined with her involvement in the Protestant faith, led her to "a day of change which would profoundly affect all the days to follow" (p. 5). It took place at a churchwomen's meeting. A Protestant missionary, Dr. Frank Laubach, whose humanitarian work and writings inspired Bonny, was scheduled to speak that evening. Earlier, he had heard her rehearsing with her accompanist for an upcoming violin performance. "You play as if God speaks through your violin," Laubach commented. And so he invited Bonny to play during the evening service. That evening, she noticed his bowed head as she began playing and recalled his comment. She later recounted:

> It was as if the violin was not my own; bow arm and fingers were held in abeyance/obedience to a light and wonderful infusion that created an unbelievable sound. … The notes mellowed and soared with exquisite grace. … I was trembling when I finished, and as I sat down, I began to shake even more violently (Bonny, 2002a, pp. 5–6).

Despite this, with the support, encouragement, and presence of Dr. Laubach, she was able to perform again, this time even more beautifully.

> Awake all night, it wasn't until morning that I found a word to describe what I was experiencing. Conversion. But with music? I had not heard of that! But it was true. I looked at the world around me in a different way: colors, forms, sounds, sensations took on a depth of dimension. I awoke early each morning singing, and seemed to float through the days. The very act of life and breath was a joy (Bonny, 2002a, p. 6)!

In the years that followed, Bonny meditated on her changed sense of self and reached out to others (Bonny, 2002a). This brought experiences of grace and new revelations about her inner self and about being alive. Along with the beauty and joy of opening up came the difficult aspects, facing what was unresolved from her past, and the struggles that lay ahead. When she needed help navigating the troubles that emerged from within her self, Bonny sought a therapist. She found that particularly someone trained in the humanistic tradition, one that supported self-actualization, intuition, emotions, and developing a clearer sense of perception, suited her needs. The therapist whom she found also practiced hypnosis. Although she would not integrate them for another ten years, by this time the fundamental elements of her method were present in her experience.

> The epiphany experience had opened the doors of my mind to a new experience with music. The reliving of early trauma through imagery processes ... had convinced me of the power of consciousness exploration. With these convictions in mind, at age 40 I applied for study in the field of music therapy (Bonny, 2002a, p. 7).

A few years after completing her music therapy training, Bonny joined the staff at the Maryland Psychiatric Research Center (MPRC) (Bonny, 2002a). At that time, the mid- to late 1960s, government-approved research was being conducted at the MPRC on the clinical uses of mind-altering drugs with persons suffering from neurosis, substance abuse, or terminal cancer. As a subject's consciousness expanded under the effects of the drugs, the researchers found that music helped to provide structure and direction to the experience, and Bonny was hired to help select music that was safest and most effective. After some research, she found that once the person was in a deeply altered state of consciousness, classical music worked best. Unlike the popular music that the participants tended to bring to the sessions, classical music was nonreferential and matched the pace, length, and content of their experiences, which gradually unfolded to tell the story of their inner worlds. It was during these sessions that Bonny also learned a unique set of guiding techniques that were needed to ensure that the subject's psychedelic trip was a successful therapeutic experience.

One day while she was not assisting during a drug session, Bonny spent time with the spouse of one of the subjects (Bonny, 2002b; Summer, 2002a). To give this woman a sense of what her husband was experiencing, Bonny suggested that she relax and listen to some of the same music. To Bonny's delight, the woman had an expansive imagery experience that lasted three hours. Without the use of any drugs, the music and the presence of a guide created a space wherein the listener could have an experience that resembled that of a subject in the drug study—a fantastic discovery. Moreover, there was a significant difference between the drug and nondrug experiences. Many of the subjects who took the mind-altering drugs were unable to recall significant parts of their trip. Summer (2002a) explains that the drugs stripped away the subject's sense of self and revealed deeper truths with which he or she was ill-prepared to cope. Whether it was a repressed memory, a deep feeling, or a hidden intention, subjects were unable to integrate what surfaced, and when the physiological impact of the drug wore off, these thoughts were once again repressed. Bonny's music-only participant was easily able to recall her experiences "because the music only elicited material that the subject was willing and ready to remember" (Summer, 2002a, p. 51). Therefore, the music was safer than the drugs because it did not penetrate too deeply and helped participants to access material that they could manage and integrate once they returned to a normal state of consciousness.

A second significant event occurred when Hanscarl Leuner, the creator of Guided Affective Imagery (GAI), visited the center and presented on his use of music in his practice (Bonny, 2002b; Summer, 2002c). Bonny volunteered to be his subject during a demonstration and found the imagery and feelings raised by the music to be profound. She later reported realizing immediately that his induction did not work well with the music that he used. In the same moments, "[a]n 'aha' experience brought the realization that somehow [she] intuitively knew how to program music to explore deep inner spaces" (Bonny, 2002a, p. 13). By this time, all of the elements were in place, and she began to craft the individual method that she named "Guided Imagery and Music."

In the early 1970s, Bonny (2002c) also began to explore the use of music imaging in an altered state of consciousness with groups of people. The first experience involved her and a group of family members who were snowbound and unable to attend church. Bonny suggested that they lie down and listen to music together instead. Before the music began, she helped them to relax and invited them to let the music lead them on an inner journey. She used a series of six pieces which she had chosen to accompany some of Leuner's ten standard imagery situations: specifically, the meadow; exploring a house as the symbol of the person; following a brook upstream to its source; following a brook downstream to the ocean; climbing a mountain and describing the view; and returning to normal consciousness. Even though she did not inform the listeners about the imagery scenes, several of them experienced these images during the corresponding music. This was another unexpected discovery. Bonny learned more as she tested her approach to group music imaging in more structured settings. She experimented with the use of programs similar to the one she had used with her family, with more structured guiding and with a verbal suggestion of the scene for each piece. She tried more sequenced programs that could facilitate spontaneous imaging for the entire experience. For these experiences, only one suggestion was used to set the listener's entire music imaging experience in motion: "Let the music take you wherever you need to go" (Bonny, 2002c, p. 62). Bonny tested programs of differing lengths. She learned to assess the listener's motivations, attention spans, and depth of relaxation prior to the music. Listeners with high motivation, openness, and attention benefited more from spontaneous imaging to longer programs. For those with shorter attention spans, greater anxiety, and less responsiveness, shorter programs and a more structured approach to guiding proved more effective. Bonny's experiments with groups thus furthered the development of her more refined individual method.

The use of 30- to 50-minute music programs in individual GIM is a unique and defining feature of Bonny's method (Bruscia, 2002a). During her work at MRPC, Bonny began designing classical music programs to facilitate the subjects' drug sessions, which lasted about 12 hours. Around the same time, she began to develop shorter programs, 30 to 40 minutes in length, in collaboration with Daniel Brown, the director of a drug counseling center (Grocke, 2002). Brown's center specialized in serving people from the community who were actively experiencing a bad trip or who were having a flashback of a prior negative experience of taking psychedelic drugs (Bonny, 2002c). Together they designed music programs for crisis intervention that covered five main areas: establishing rapport, generating guided imagery, encouraging emotional expression and release, processing through the terminal stages of the session, and facilitating positive experiences.

Later in the 1970s, Bonny worked toward a Ph.D. and further developed her ability to program music by focusing her doctoral work on the development of 12 programs (Bonny, 2002a). Her dissertation included a structural analysis of the music she selected for the programs, an analysis of the "inner morphology" or potential effect on the listener, and a theoretical basis for the clinical use of music programs in altered-states work. Bonny (2002d) used the stages of the psychedelic drug experience (pre-onset, onset, build to peak, peak, stabilization, return) that she identified while working at MRPC as a guide for selecting and sequencing pieces. The 12 programs were titled: Group Experience, Imagery, Quiet Music, Comforting/Anaclytic, Nurturing, Mostly Bach, Emotional Expression I, Peak Experience, Positive Affect, Transitions, Affect Release, and Death/Rebirth (Bonny, 2002d). Whereas each program represents a unique soundscape, program titles such as "Relationships," "Peak Experience," and "Death/Rebirth" are merely suggestive; they are not "accurate predictors of specific imagery, emotional processes, imager reactions, or therapeutic outcomes" (Bruscia, 2002c, p. 307).

In her final design, the individual GIM session lasts 1½ to 2 hours, though there are extraordinary situations when, due to client need, a session can last up to 3 hours. Instead of the titles *therapist* and *client*, Bonny came to refer to the therapist as the *guide* and to the client as the *traveler*. These terms are used interchangeably throughout this study.

A GIM session consists of four phases: Prelude (20–30 min.), Induction (10–15 min.), Music Experience (30–50 min.), and Postlude (20–30 min.). During the Prelude, the therapist uses a nondirective approach to assist the client in exploration of important issues, concerns, or goals. This exploration can be verbal (therapist–client dialogue) and/or nonverbal (most often mandala drawing). The Induction is a time for the guide to help the traveler to relax, focus inward, and prepare to engage theme(s) that emerged during the Prelude. The induction usually culminates with the guide presenting the traveler with a starting image. In GIM, imagery experiences include sensations, emotions, memories, and fantasies. As the music begins and the music experience unfolds, the therapist engages the client in reporting his or her experience and offers support, guidance, and assistance to help the client fully access and work through what emerges. The therapist also maintains a written transcript of the verbal dialogue and significant events. During the music experience, the guide does not direct the traveler's experience. Instead, the guide accompanies the traveler as they both open to the music and to what emerges from the traveler's experience of it. Guiding interventions are mostly verbal, but there are times when physical interventions may be helpful. Before using any physical interventions, the therapist informs the client and asks her or his permission to proceed. During the Postlude, the guide helps the traveler to integrate the experience and explore their meaning and relevance to current life.

Expansion and Development of the GIM Method

During the following two decades, GIM spread around the world, and the clinical applications and permutations of the method widened (Bonny & Goldberg, 2002; Bruscia, 2002a, 2002c; Clark, 2002; Grocke, 2002c; Lewis, 2002; Summer, 2002c). Mostly used in private settings to help individual adults with anxiety, depression, loss, life transitions, and self-actualization, individual and Group GIM practices grew to include persons in psychiatric (Blake & Bishop, 1994; Booth, 2005–2006; Goldberg, 1994; Summer, 1988) and medical (Pickett, 1996–1997; Short, 2002; Wigle-Justice & Kasayka, 1999) hospitals, substance abuse programs (Moe, 2011–2012; Murphy, 2008; Skaggs, 1997a), hospices (Marr, 1998–1999), and nursing homes (Short, 1992, 1997; Summer, 1981) and with a wide variety of illnesses and disorders (Burns, 2002; Clarkson, 1995; Goldberg, Hoss, & Chesna, 1988; Hahna & Borling, 2002–2004; Meadows, 2002; Moe, Roesen, & Raben, 2000; Short, 2002). GIM was also used with children and adolescents (Powell, 2007–2008; Roy, 1996–1997; Skaggs, 1997b; Wesley, 2002). Some practitioners combined GIM with other approaches (Blake, 1994; Booth, 2005–2006; Clarkson, 2002; Holligan, 1994; Pickett & Sonnen, 1993), and others moved outside of the humanistic tradition and applied other theoretical orientations to GIM (Bruscia, 1995, 2002b; Summer, 1998; Ward, 2002). Along with this rapid expansion came adaptations to the method. Parallel to this growth, imagery techniques both with and without music were being developed outside of the GIM community, and oftentimes these were referred to as *Guided Imagery* (Bruscia, 2002a). In response to this, in 1996 Bonny decided to change the name of her method from Guided Imagery and Music to the *Bonny Method of Guided Imagery and Music*.

CHAPTER TWO

THE MAIN COMPONENTS OF GIM AND THE BONNY METHOD

The Association for Music and Imagery (AMI), the professional association for GIM fellows, defines the Bonny Method of Guided Imagery and Music as:

> [A] music-assisted transformational therapy that offers persons the opportunity to integrate mental, emotional, physical, and spiritual aspects of themselves....[It] is characterized by the use of specially sequenced western classical music designed to stimulate and sustain a dynamic unfolding of imagery experiences. Sessions in this one-to-one modality are conducted by facilitators who are formally trained in The Bonny Method of GIM (Association for Music and Imagery, 2010).

According to the AMI (2010) training standards, GIM training is focused on the individual form of Bonny Method; however, the specific practices that constitute the method are neither clearly specified nor differentiated from the practices that have been developed by Bonny's proponents or from the practices that fall outside of the realm of GIM. The developments inside and outside of the GIM community during the past few decades raise the need to address the following questions: What specifically constitutes the practice of the Bonny Method of Guided Imagery and Music? What constitutes an adaptation of the Bonny Method? What should these adapted practices be called? What about group sessions? What are they called? Are group practices adaptations of the practices used in individual (one-to-one) sessions? What practices does the term "Guided Imagery and Music" represent? To date, no consensus has been reached among GIM practitioners regarding what defines the individual and group forms of the Bonny Method, what adaptations to it are acceptable, and what names should be applied to these adaptations. So, why is it important to answer these questions? Bruscia (2002a) has addressed this directly:

> [These] practices vary considerably in goal, technique, orientation, and process, yet they are often confused with one another, causing a lack of conceptual clarity in the work itself, as well as misunderstandings about the competence requirements for practitioners. This in turn raises serious issues about the ethics of the safe practice of GIM. Who is competent to do what kinds of work, and what kinds of training are necessary to practice the various techniques combining music, expanded states of consciousness, or imagery (p. 39)?

Bruscia (2002a) has tackled these issues and presented a cogent set of definitions that establish clear boundaries for these various practices. Before presenting these, it will be helpful to describe the nomenclature as presented by Bruscia. Note that the terms *modification* and *adaptation* are used interchangeably in this study.

According to Bruscia (2002a), Guided Imagery and Music (GIM) is a general title that includes all of the individual and group practices that Bonny created, all modifications of these practices, and all of the forms of imaging to music in an altered state of consciousness that her work inspired. In contrast, the title, the Bonny Method, refers to *both* the individual and group forms of GIM specifically developed by Bonny, and the full title, the Bonny Method of Guided Imagery and Music, and its acronym (BMGIM) refer *only* to the individual method created by Bonny. The title *Group GIM* refers to Bonny's group form. Therefore, in this study, practices that represent modifications of Bonny's individual or group work are simply referred to as GIM.

Sometimes it is the alteration of a thing that brings its key features into sharp focus and brings new understandings (Bonny & Goldberg, 2002). Adaptations to the Bonny Method brought the need to clarify what Bonny created, to identify the parts of her method that can be modified, and to clarify the boundary between GIM and other imagery practices involving music. Such boundaries are essential. They provided a clear dividing line between practices that were included and those that were excluded from the survey, and they highlight and clearly define the variables of practice that are important and need to be treated as distinct. To define the boundaries of GIM and the Bonny Method, Bruscia (2002a) compared and differentiated these practices in terms of the following variables: states of consciousness, spontaneous imaging, use of classical music programs, goals, theoretical orientation, verbal dialogue, and length of session and music.

What follows is a summary of the distinctions presented by Bruscia (2002a). This summary describes the practices that define the Bonny Method and the boundaries between it and other GIM practices and between GIM and music therapy techniques that involve imaging to music. GIM practices referred to in this section that fall outside the boundaries of the Bonny Method but are included in the survey are described in greater detail in Chapters Three through Seven. All of the Bonny Method practices described in the current chapter are included in the survey.

State of Consciousness

In individual or group sessions designed by Bonny, the traveler listens to music in an expanded state of consciousness, and then, within this environment, the traveler further explores consciousness. According to Bruscia (2002a), the same holds for all GIM work: "Only those music listening experiences that occur within an expanded state of consciousness fall within the boundaries of GIM" (p. 48). For instance, during a typical *music relaxation* experience, a technique commonly used in music therapy, the combination of the music and the therapist's verbal directions is used to help the client to achieve and maintain a state of relaxation. In GIM, the therapist's verbal direction is aimed at helping the traveler achieve a relaxed state which in turn helps to further open or expand his or her state of consciousness during the subsequent music listening. In music relaxation, the purpose is to relax the conscious mind, not to open, expand, or explore consciousness.

In *projective listening*, another technique used in music therapy, expansion of consciousness is limited further as the clients sit upright and listen in an ordinary state of consciousness. Moreover, in projective listening, the client is asked to "identify, describe, interpret, and/or free associate" to music, not to openly explore consciousness within the music (Bruscia, 1998a, p. 124).

Spontaneous Imaging

In BMGIM or Group GIM sessions, the traveler enters an expanded state and explores consciousness by *freely and spontaneously* imaging to music (Bruscia, 2002a). After the guide offers a starting image, from which the traveler is free to move away, the images come solely from the traveler's consciousness while in direct contact with the music. During the music, if the guide limits the client's freedom by offering images, or by directing the traveler's imaging, the guide is no longer practicing the Bonny Method and may not even be practicing GIM. Bruscia (2002a) refers to three types of spontaneous imaging, other than the free type: (1) contained spontaneous imaging, (2) directed imaging, and (3) re-imaging.

In *contained spontaneous music imaging*, the guide provides an image to be used for the entire experience and periodically provides suggestions to move the traveler from one location to another for exploration. In other words, the traveler's spontaneous imaging is contained within an image that is provided by the guide (e.g., a house); the traveler's spontaneous imaging does not emerge freely in relation to the music. Therefore, contained spontaneous imaging is GIM but not the Bonny Method.

In the second type, *directed music imaging*, there is no free exploration of consciousness. Instead, the therapist leads the client through an imagery experience by providing images for the client step by step, thus severely limiting the client's freedom to image freely and spontaneously to the music. In other words, the images are produced by the therapist, and the client's imaging is directed by the therapist. Therefore, directed music imaging is not the Bonny Method or GIM at all, but a music therapy technique.

The third type, *re-imaging*, involves a shortened GIM session wherein the traveler freely and spontaneously explores the imagery experience of another person. The other person's image (e.g., a fellow client, a loved one, etc.) is presented as the starting image, but unlike in a BMGIM session, the traveler commits to exploring that image during the music. Bruscia (2002a) notes that re-imaging is a sort of contained imaging in that the traveler freely explores his or her consciousness within the context of someone else's image, yet unlike in contained spontaneous imaging, the guide does not introduce or direct imagery during the music. Like contained spontaneous imaging, re-imaging is GIM but not the Bonny Method because the imagery focus does not emerge from the client's free and spontaneous imaging to the music.

State of Consciousness and Spontaneous Imaging

In summary, the Bonny Method involves listening to music while in an expanded state of consciousness and further exploring consciousness within the music (Bruscia, 2002a). In the Bonny Method, clients image freely and spontaneously to the music. Other types of spontaneous imaging (e.g., contained spontaneous imaging and re-imaging) fall outside the boundaries of the Bonny Method because the clients do not image freely for the entire music experience or solely within the context of images produced by them during the music. These techniques are still considered GIM because they involve the client imaging spontaneously to music for the purpose of expanding and exploring of consciousness. Though contained spontaneous imaging and re-imaging have an impact on the expansion and exploration of consciousness, their purpose is to focus consciousness, not to limit it. Practices that do not involve the expansion and exploration of consciousness (e.g., music relaxation, projective listening, directed music imaging) fall outside the boundaries of GIM practice.

Classical Music Programs

Bonny chose classical music for use in individual sessions because she found it to be the optimal type of music for expanding and exploring consciousness. In her words, "classical selections are able to provide depth of experience, variety of color and form, [and] harmonic and melodic complexity which are qualities needed for self-exploration" (Bonny, 2002e, p. 150). Moreover, she carefully selected pieces of classical music and grouped and sequenced them into programs lasting 30 to 50 minutes. "Each program was given its own affective contour, sensitively timed to lead the traveler into a particular state of consciousness and/or emotional space, hold the traveler there, and then provide a pathway back out" (Bruscia, 2002a, p. 56). In the Bonny Method, the guide carefully chooses a program to facilitate the client's work and allows the client's experience to unfold without interrupting the music. In contrast, some GIM therapists practice what can be called *spontaneous programming*. Instead of selecting a program and allowing it to run its course, the spontaneous programmer follows the client and changes the music in response to the client's unfolding experience (Ventre, 2002). This can involve moving from one program to another or selecting individual pieces and sequencing them extemporaneously. Originally, this involved moving between tracks within one vinyl record album or reel-to-reel tape or from one album or tape to another. As the technology developed, it involved moving within or between cassette tapes, then compact discs (Bruscia, 2002c), and, more recently, digital files (e.g., .wav, .aiff, .flac, .mp3).

Bonny's use of music in Group GIM was more varied (Bruscia, 2002a). Group GIM sessions included classical or nonclassical music, and predesigned programs were an option alongside whatever single selection or combination of selections suited the group format and the needs and goals of the participants.

In summary, a defining feature of the BMGIM (the individual form) is the use of entire predesigned programs of classical music (Bruscia, 2002a). When the guide engages in spontaneous programming or when nonclassical music is used in individual sessions, the practice falls outside the boundaries of the Bonny Method. The use of predesigned programs and the use of classical music is not a defining feature of Group GIM.

Goals

Throughout her writings, Bonny referred to both therapeutic and nontherapeutic goals of GIM. This was probably due to her humanistic and spiritual orientation and her different experiences working in both individual and group settings, which will be discussed in the next section.

Bruscia (2002a) points out that Bonny's fondness for humanistic psychology can make it unclear whether her goals for individual and group work were therapeutic.

> In the humanistic orientation, health is emphasized over pathology, and the primary goal of all work, whether called therapy or not, is self-actualization … . Consequently, even when Bonny worked with individuals within a clear psychotherapeutic framework, the goals were characteristically holistic, growth-oriented, and transpersonal rather than pathology-driven and purely psychological (pp. 47–48).

Bonny's (2002f) interest in spirituality and transpersonal psychology also invites ambiguity. The terms *spirituality* and *transpersonal* seem to express a similar if not the same concept. Bonny stated:

> Spirituality is the personal act or process of transformation that takes one from an ego-centered, exclusionary attitude toward life to one filled with inclusionary attitudes of love, acceptance, adoration, appreciation for all life forms, a sense of unity and purpose that extends into the past and into the future (Bonny, 2002f, p. 179).

According to Abrams (2002), transpersonal experiences "transcend the usual scope of individual human identity, personality and ego, encompass the wider aspects of humankind, life, the psyche, and the cosmos, and transcend limits of space and time" (p. 104). Goals formulated from within a spiritual or transpersonal orientation, which are well suited to the types of music experiences that travelers have in GIM, do not preclude psychological outcomes, but they do not assure them either (Kasayka, 2002). Though spirituality was very important to Bonny, she wrote little about it (Kasayka, 2002; Summer, 2002b). When referring to therapeutic work, she favored the term *transpersonal*, reserving the term *spiritual* for nontherapeutic work (Bruscia, 2002a) despite the similar nature of these types of experiences in the music.

In reviewing her writings regarding differences between individual and group work, Bruscia (2002a) found that Bonny consistently referred to her work using individual GIM as music psychotherapy with therapeutic goals for the client. In contrast, he found that her goals for Group GIM were nontherapeutic (i.e., educational, spiritual, personal growth). Through her early experimentation, Bonny discovered that the traveler-guide dyad in individual GIM was the "primary and most effective mode of exploration into the deeper unconscious" (2002e, p. 147). On the other hand, the experiences that people had during the group sessions seemed to Bonny (2002e) "peripheral by comparison" (p. 147). Therefore, therapeutic goals were frequently adopted for individual BMGIM sessions, but not as frequently adopted for Group GIM.

A further complication of this distinction between individual and group work is that there is some disagreement as to whether Bonny created a form of GIM for groups at all. Summer (2002c) argues that Group GIM is a misnomer for several reasons. In Bonny's group sessions, there was no guiding during the music experience and, as Summer points out, facilitating deep individual process in a group setting can be antithetical to the goal of facilitating group processes. In addition, Bonny did not experiment with or develop her group format for use in clinical contexts to address clinical goals.

This work was done by GIM practitioners who followed her and who also happened to be music therapists. For this and other reasons, Summer argues that this type of work is a practice belonging to music therapy and should be referred to as *Group Music and Imagery Therapy*, not Group GIM. Bruscia (2002a) and Summer (2002c) do agree that distinguishing between Bonny's nontherapeutic work with groups and the therapeutic work of her proponents is important. As stated earlier, for this study, Bonny's group form is referred to as Group GIM, and clinical applications are referred to as GIM.

In summary, though she advocated for therapeutic and nontherapeutic uses of both individual and Group GIM, "Bonny did not work extensively with nor did she develop methodological principles for using the *individual form* for *nontherapeutic* purposes; likewise, she did not work extensively with nor did she develop methodological principles for using the *group form* for *therapeutic* purposes" (Bruscia, 2002a, p. 48). The individual form of the Bonny Method is defined by having therapeutic goals; in contrast, the use of the individual form to address nontherapeutic goals falls outside of the Bonny Method. The group form of the Bonny Method is defined by having nontherapeutic goals; in contrast, the use of the group form to address therapeutic goals falls outside of the Bonny Method.

Theoretical Orientation

The individual and group forms of the Bonny Method are defined by a humanistic or transpersonal approach; the use of other theoretical orientations constitutes a modification of the Bonny Method (Bruscia, 2002a). Therefore, any use of the individual or group form within a psychodynamic, cognitive-behavioral, or other theoretical framework goes beyond the boundaries of the Bonny Method as originally conceived by Bonny and therefore falls under the generic category of GIM.

Verbal Dialogue

In the individual BMGIM session, the guide initiates and maintains a verbal dialogue with the traveler during the music imaging experience. This continuous dialoguing with the client during the music experience defines the individual form of the Bonny Method. Therefore, if there is no dialogue during the music imaging, but the rest of the session structure is unchanged, the practice is GIM, but not the Bonny Method (Bruscia, 2002a).

In a typical Group GIM session, the guide does not initiate and maintain a verbal dialogue with the travelers during the music experience; rather, they image alone without intervention from the therapist (Bruscia, 2002a). When there is no dialogue during group music imaging and the rest of the session structure is unchanged, the practice is the Bonny Method. When there is an active dialogue among and between the group and guide during the music imaging, the practice is GIM, but not the Bonny method (Bruscia, 2002a). Several types of group sessions that include verbal dialogue during the music have been developed by Bonny's proponents. Some involve dialogue between the travelers, some are guided by the therapist, and some involve a combination of both. These adaptations are detailed in Chapter Five.

Directive Interventions

Another adaptation occurs when the guide responds to the traveler's spontaneous imaging with directive interventions. Directive interventions are verbal comments by the guide that tell the traveler what to do. These kinds of directive interventions are not part of the Bonny Method and therefore, when used in the individual or group form, are considered to be GIM, not the Bonny Method. It should also be noted that directive interventions in response to the client's spontaneous imaging are different from "directed music imaging," which as described earlier, involves actually dictating what the client images, which is not a GIM practice.

The issue of directiveness is related to theoretical orientation. According to Bruscia, directive guiding interventions are most often borrowed from other treatment methods or orientations (e.g., energetic, Gestalt, cognitive), and they are used to achieve therapeutic outcomes that emanate from outside of the client's spontaneous imaging. In a humanistic approach, the aim is to focus on the client's experience and to allow solutions to emerge from within the client and from within the context of the client's worldview. Thus any sort of directive guiding is not part of the Bonny Method.

Going one step further, in the Bonny Method, all of the guide's interventions within every phase of the session are formulated from within a humanistic or transpersonal orientation which is characteristically nondirective. However, when the guide uses only nondirective interventions during the music imaging but formulates them from within another orientation (e.g., behavioral, psychodynamic), the practice is not the Bonny Method. Likewise, when the guide intervenes verbally during the prelude and postlude from within another orientation, the practice is not the Bonny Method.

As a point of clarification, guiding can include both verbal interventions and physical interventions (e.g., holding the client's hand, holding a pillow for the client to hit, cradling the client's neck, etc.). Verbal and physical interventions can also be considered directive or nondirective in approach. Bonny's Method (2002g) includes the nondirective use of physical interventions. Specifically, in the Bonny Method, the guide typically asks the traveler for permission to physically intervene or even asks the traveler what kind of physical intervention may be needed. These nondirective physical interventions are used only in response to the client's experience of the music and only when they are clearly indicated (e.g., the client reports being disoriented and cannot get reoriented without the therapist's help).

In summary, the Bonny Method involves dialogue between guide and traveler during the music in individual sessions, but no dialogue during group sessions. During BMGIM sessions, the therapist uses nondirective interventions during the prelude, music imaging, and postlude that are formulated from within a humanistic or transpersonal orientation. Nondirective interventions that are formulated from within a psychodynamic, cognitive-behavioral, or other theoretical orientation may be considered GIM, but not the Bonny Method. Individual GIM sessions that include directive verbal interventions during the prelude, music imaging, and postlude are beyond the Bonny Method.

Length of Session and Music Experience

As described earlier, the individual session that Bonny designed typically lasts 1½ to 2 hours, and in some cases up to 3 hours. For reasons that are covered in Chapter Three, individual GIM sessions may be shortened to less than 1½ hours. Shortened sessions preclude use of 30- to 50-minute music programs, the type designed by Bonny. With a shorter program, there is less time for music to develop and for the journey to unfold, and this lessens the client's potential for expansion and exploration of consciousness (Bruscia, 2002a). In addition, with an overall shorter session, the guide is compelled to ensure that the depth of the client's music experience is commensurate with the length and utility of the shortened music program and the time available to process it afterward. Therefore, shortened individual GIM sessions are a modification of the Bonny Method.

Group GIM sessions by Bonny in nonclinical settings as well as sessions with groups in clinical settings have varied in length and the amount of music used depending on the goals and needs of the group (Bruscia, 2002a). Group sessions of either type may last 1 to 1½ hours, with the music imaging portion ranging from 3 to 20 minutes, and the prelude, induction, and postlude adjusted to suit (Bonny, 2002e; Bruscia, 2002a). Therefore, GIM sessions for groups can vary considerably in length without being considered a modification of the Bonny Method. Note that within the context of this study this distinction is for the most part moot because most of the work using Group GIM is in clinical contexts with therapeutic goals and thus falls outside the Bonny Method. In other words, GIM work with groups for therapeutic purposes represents a modification in terms of goals but not in terms of length of session and music.

Summary

The individual and group forms of the Bonny Method have been defined and differentiated from the modifications that followed Bonny's pioneering work (Bruscia, 2002a). According to Bruscia (2002a), the individual form of the Bonny Method or BMGIM is defined as "a modality of therapy involving spontaneous imaging, expanded states of consciousness, predesigned classical music programs, ongoing dialogues during the music-imaging, and nondirective guiding techniques" (p. 59). Bonny's group form, referred to as Group GIM, is defined as "a modality for self-development involving spontaneous imaging, expanded states, various styles of music selected by the guide, and no dialogues or guiding during the music-imaging" (Bruscia, 2002a, p. 59).

GIM practices that fall outside the boundaries of the Bonny Method include spontaneous imaging within images that are presented by the therapist during the induction (e.g., re-imaging) and spontaneous imaging within images that are presented by the therapist during the music (e.g., contained spontaneous imaging); formulating interventions (directive or nondirective) from other than a humanistic or transpersonal orientation; directive guiding of spontaneous music imaging; the shortening of individual sessions; the use of spontaneous programming and nonclassical music during individual sessions; and dialogue during group sessions.

Music therapy practices that do not include expansion and exploration of consciousness through the client's spontaneous imaging to music (e.g., relaxation listening, projective listening, and directed music imaging) fall outside the boundaries of the Bonny Method and of GIM. These distinctions between the Bonny Method, modifications, and non-GIM (Bruscia, 2002a) are outlined in Table 1 and Table 2.

Table 1

Bonny's Individual Form and Modifications

	Individual GIM		Not GIM
	Bonny Method	Modification	
Consciousness	Expand and Explore		Ordinary
			Relaxed
Imaging	Free and Spontaneous	Contained Spontaneous	Directed
		Re-imaging	
Music	Classical	Nonclassical	
Programming	Predesigned	Extemporaneous	
Goals	Therapeutic	Nontherapeutic	
Orientation	Humanistic, Transpersonal/ Spiritual	Psychodynamic, Jungian, etc.	
Dialogue	Nondirective	Directive	
		No Dialogue	
Length (Session)	1½–2 hours	1 hour or less	
Length (Music)	30–50 minutes	Less than 30 minutes	

Table 2

Bonny's Group Form and Modifications

	Group GIM		Not GIM
	Bonny Method	Modification	
Consciousness	Expand and Explore		Ordinary
			Relaxed
Imaging	Free and Spontaneous	Contained Spontaneous	Directed
		Re-imaging	
Music	Varied		
Programming	Varied		
Goals	Nontherapeutic	Therapeutic	
Orientation	Humanistic, Transpersonal/ Spiritual	Psychodynamic, Jungian, etc.	
Dialogue	No Dialogue	Dialogue	
Length (Session)	Varied		
Length (Music)	Varied		

CHAPTER THREE

VARIATIONS IN LENGTH OF SESSION AND MUSIC

In Chapters Three through Six, results from the survey of GIM fellows (Muller, 2010) will be presented, followed by a review of the literature on Bonny Method practices and modifications. The 2010 survey data will be presented in lay terms, but represent results that were statistically significant. Each chapter covers data and literature related to specific components of practice, namely: length of session and music; selection and use of music; verbal dialogue and guiding; and theoretical orientation. Other components of practice, consciousness, imaging, and goals, will be used to further delineate boundaries. Each chapter section will include a brief summary and discussion.

The individual Bonny Method session is defined by a 1½- to 2-hour or longer session with a music listening portion that lasts 30 minutes or longer (Bruscia, 2002). Group GIM is not defined in terms of session length or amount of music, and both can vary greatly without being considered a modification of the Bonny Method.

Most Frequent Practices

Because Group GIM can vary so widely and still be within the boundaries of the Bonny Method, the survey research was focused on contemporary practices in individual work. In responding to the survey, practitioners indicated how frequently they used a practice (e.g., 1½- to 2-hour session) using a Likert scale (never, seldom, sometimes, often, always). The results related to length of session and music are summarized below. The percentages represent the sum of all practitioners' ratings for a given practice, with the total ratings across the Likert scale adding up to 100%. For example, the standard 1½ - to 2-hour individual session with 30+-minute music portions was still being used often or always by most practitioners (82%); thus 18% were using this sometimes, seldom, or never. One-hour sessions were used often or sometimes by many practitioners (65%); ½-hour sessions were used seldom or never. For standard-length sessions, shorter music portions were also being used. Twenty-one to 30 minutes of music was used often or sometimes (80%) and 11–20 minutes was used sometimes or less often (88%), while 6–10 minutes and 1–5 minutes were used seldom or never by most practitioners (88%). For sessions lasting less than 1½–2 hours, 21–30, 11–20, and 6–10 minutes of music were used often or sometimes by 60% to 70% of practitioners, while 1–5 minutes was used sometimes or less by 70%.

In summary, as of 2010, shortened session lengths and music imaging portions were in use by GIM fellows, but much less frequently than the Bonny Method standard, with perhaps two exceptions: the use of 21–30 minutes of music during a 1½- to 2-hour session and the use of a 1-hour session. Twenty-one to 30 minutes of music during a 1½- to 2-hour session was being used nearly as much as more than 30 minutes of music. In the author's experience, it is standard practice for a GIM fellow to skip a single piece(s) within a full-length program or to fade the program out prior to its completion. This is done even for the most psychologically stable client when a shorter or less intense travel is indicated during a BMGIM session. Bruscia (2003) has discussed the type of decision-making involved in eliminating pieces from full-length programs and has made some recommendations for this with regard to specific music programs. In addition, a number of programs have been designed for use in GIM sessions that last 21–30 minutes (Bruscia & Grocke, 2002). In terms of modifications to GIM practice, perhaps the use of 21–30 minutes of music during a 1½- to 2-hour session is a minimal one. The other exception, the use of a 1-hour session, may not be considered a minimal modification because it requires modifications to every other phase of the session.

The survey revealed that GIM fellows who practice outside the United States use a 1½- to 2-hour session more often than those practicing within the United States. This may be explained by differences in health care delivery systems inside and outside the United States. Cultural differences regarding individual therapy

Variations in Length of Session and Music

inside and outside the United States might also provide an explanation for this difference.

A comparison of session length and music length with age and populations served indicates that some of them may vary in relation to each other. It is important to note here that a type of statistical procedure known as a correlation was recalculated for this book. In technical terms, the Pearson product-moment correlation coefficient which was used in the survey to calculate corelationships between specific practices and the age and populations served is best suited for ratio data. In the survey data, these practitioner frequency ratings were not in fact ratio data, but instead ordinal data. The mistake was made because frequency ratings (never, seldom, sometimes, often, always) were recoded to digits (1, 2, 3, 4, 5) to allow the statistical software to perform calculations, and this made the data appear to statisticians as ratio in nature. A test known as Spearman's rank correlation coefficient, which is better suited for ordinal data, was used to recalculate the correlations for presentation in this book. Comparison of practitioner frequency ratings of session length and music length with ratings of age and populations served revealed that those who more often worked with adolescents also tended to use ½-hour sessions more often, while they used 1½- to 2-hour sessions less often; conversely, those who more frequently worked with well-adults tended to use 1½-hour sessions more often but ½-hour sessions less often. Practitioners who worked more frequently with normal neurosis tended to use 6–10 and 21–30 minutes of music during 1½- to 2-hour sessions more frequently, while those who worked with trauma survivors more often tended to use 1–5 minutes of music during a less-than-1½-hour session more often. Practitioners who more frequently worked with older adults tended to use shorter segments of music (1–5 minutes) within the standard 1½- to 2-hour session length more often. These findings are consistent with the literature on work with client age groups and clinical concerns, which are covered in the next section.

Specific Practices

The clinical literature on GIM provides many insights into why and how the length of an individual session and its music listening portion are modified. The literature also provides insights into the length variations in group sessions. The discussion of the literature has been organized into four main groups of clientele: psychiatric, physical illness, elderly, and children.

Psychiatric

GIM practitioners have reported the use of shorter sessions and shorter music imaging portions for adult clients with adjustment disorder, depression, anxiety, posttraumatic stress disorder (PTSD), drug and alcohol addiction, personality disorder, schizophrenia, and autism. In private practice settings, Summer (1998) and Summer and Chong (2006) have reduced music imaging to only one or two pieces of music during full-length individual GIM sessions. Clarkson (1995) used 60-minute GIM sessions that included 5–20 minutes of music imaging for a nonverbal man with autism. These three authors used these modifications to limit the depth of the client's experience, i.e., to decrease the potential for expansion and exploration of consciousness. In contrast, Ritchey Vaux (1993) has written about the application of GIM within a 50-minute session to make scheduling more manageable in her psychotherapy practice. In this format, the prelude and induction last no more than 15 minutes combined, and the music imaging no more than 20 minutes, leaving 10–15 minutes for postlude processing. This author stressed the importance of preparing clients for the shortened session by explaining the need to move swiftly from discussion to music as well as the need for them to further process and integrate the music experience on their own as there was merely time in the session to review images.

Shortened overall sessions or shorter music imaging segments were generally recommended for psychiatric clients who have an impaired sense of self (ego) (Wrangsjö, 1994). For example, institutionalized psychiatric clients typically experience a decrease in ego strength; therefore, limiting the depth of the music imaging can be imperative (Summer, 1988). In psychiatric settings, Goldberg (1994) has limited the music imaging during individual sessions to 15–30 minutes, whereas Summer (1988) has limited entire GIM sessions to 30 minutes.

Several authors offered general recommendations for shortening the music imaging portion of sessions for traumatized individuals (Hahna & Borling, 2003–2004; Korlin, 2002; Moffitt & Hall, 2003–2004) to minimize the evocation of traumatic imagery (Korlin, 2002) and to accommodate traumatized clients who have sensitivities to sound (Moffitt & Hall, 2003–2004). Shorter music programs were also indicated for work with individual hospitalized patients diagnosed with PTSD (Blake, 1994; Blake & Bishop, 1994).

All of the shortened sessions and music listening portions described above constitute modifications of the BMGIM. Whether the purpose is to accommodate client need or scheduling, when there is less time for music listening, there is less potential for expansion and exploration of consciousness. A shortened prelude and induction leaves less time to help the client relax, focus, and open in preparation for the music, and a shortened postlude further compels the therapist to limit the depth of the experience (Bruscia, 2002a).

Group GIM sessions lasting 1½ hours have also been reported for inpatient psychiatric patients (Moe, Roesen, & Raben, 2000; Summer, 1988). Moe, Roesen, and Raben (2000) have used only 10 minutes of music within this time frame. Sessions can begin with a brief discussion, followed by a brief relaxation (e.g., a few deep breaths) (Goldberg, 1994; Moe, Roesen, & Raben, 2000). A shortened (1- to 2-minute) relaxation induction was recommended by Blake and Bishop (1994) when using GIM for groups of patients with PTSD. For residents of drug and alcohol treatment facilities, two authors described the use of 60-minute Group GIM sessions, with music imaging lasting from 6–8 minutes (Skaggs, 1997a) or from 5–12 minutes (Murphy, 2008), while another described the use of 90-minute sessions with 10 minutes of music (Moe, 2011–2012). For both, session length was based on facility scheduling and length of music imaging was based on the clients' readiness and the time needed to effectively prepare for and process the experience. As indicated in Chapter Two, shortened session length and music imaging in group sessions do not represent adaptations of Group GIM (Bruscia, 2002a); however, these variations in group practice are included in this book.

Physical Illness

As with psychiatric patients, adaptations have been made in this category to limit the depth of the client's experience. Wigle-Justice and Kasayka (1999) described the use of shortened individual sessions to accommodate medical patients who are physically weak or emotionally fragile, with longer-than-usual inductions and 6–15 minutes of music imaging. These authors also described Group GIM sessions with brief inductions and 10 minutes of music imaging for these same patients (Wigle-Justice & Kasayka, 1999). Marr (1998–1999) has used individual GIM within the framework of a 50-minute hour (Ritchey Vaux, 1993) for patients in end-of-life care. Her sessions included up to 15 minutes of music imaging, with brief prelude discussion and postlude processing to accommodate limited concentration due to frailty, pain, or the effects of medication (Marr, 1998–1999).

As stated above, the clinical literature reveals that modifications to the Bonny Method are based on the psychological or physical fragility of a client, but not on his or her diagnoses. Survey respondents were not queried as to the current stage of illness of their clients with cancer or terminal illness or the extent of clients' symptoms or characteristics of their psychological states. The literature supports the shortening of music listening portions of individual GIM sessions for clients who are medically fragile (Wigle-Justice & Kasayka, 1999) or in end- of-life care (Marr, 1998–1999) when sessions last less than 1½ hours, but no literature was found to support the shortening of music listening portions of full-length individual sessions solely based on diagnoses such as cancer or terminal illness.

Elderly

Summer (1981) has led group sessions with a music portion lasting up to 7 minutes with nursing home residents. Similarly, Short (1992) has used group sessions with physically disabled elderly residents that last 1 hour and music imaging portions that last 4–12 minutes. Session length was chosen to accommodate the attention span and the physical stamina of the patients, as well as facility scheduling (Short, 1992). Short (2007) offered "open" 1-hour group sessions to elderly residents. She limited the music imaging to 3–5 minutes, as some of the residents were physically and psychologically vulnerable. Again, these are not adaptations but variations in length that are included.

Children and Adolescents

Wesley (2002) has led individual sessions lasting 20 to 30 minutes with 5–10 minutes of music imaging for boys of ages 6–10 in a locked psychiatric unit. These sessions were shortened to accommodate the clients' age and their psychiatric symptoms. As with the shortened sessions for individual adults in psychiatric or medical treatment, Wesley's shortened sessions decreased the potential for expansion and exploration of consciousness and are thus adaptations of the Bonny Method.

Skaggs (1997b) has reported the use of sessions of unspecified length that revolve around imaging to a single piece of music with groups of male juvenile sex offenders in a residential treatment program. Short pieces of music were chosen to accommodate facility scheduling. Powell (2007–2008) has provided sessions lasting 5–45 minutes with music imaging lasting 3–5 minutes during music education classes with mostly high-risk children in 3rd through 8th grades. Roy (1996–1997) has used Group GIM sessions of up to 40 minutes with 5–20 minutes of music imaging during music classes with girls in a high school setting. Both Powell and Roy designed sessions to fit the scheduled class period. Like the shortening of group sessions for adult psychiatric and medical patients and for the elderly, the shortening of group sessions for children and adolescents does not constitute an adaptation of Group GIM but is included.

Summary

In summary, shortened session lengths and music imaging have been reported in the literature for use in individual sessions with psychiatric, physically ill, and child clients. Sessions and music are most often shortened to accommodate client need (fragile ego, physical frailty, limited attention span), but are also shortened to accommodate therapist or facility scheduling. Session lengths ranging from 30 to 60 minutes were reported for psychiatric clients with music listening portions lasting 5 to 30 minutes. Session lengths shorter than the standard 1½ hours but otherwise unspecified were reported for physically ill clients with music listening portions lasting 6 to 15 minutes. One exception to this was the use of the 50-minute GIM session for patients in end-of-life care. Session lengths of 20 to 30 minutes were reported for children with music portions lasting 5 to 10 minutes. The survey revealed that all of these time variations are in use.

Variations in session lengths and music imaging have also been reported for group sessions with psychiatric, physically ill, elderly, and child clients. As with individual sessions, group session length and music imaging are based on client need and facility scheduling. Group sessions for psychiatric clients range from 60 to 90 minutes with music portions lasting 5 to 12 minutes. Very brief relaxation inductions are specifically recommended for groups of patients with PTSD and those who are psychological or physical fragile as a result of physical illness. Sessions for groups of elderly patients are reported to last 60 minutes with music portions that range from 3 to 12 minutes. Group sessions for children and adolescents range from 5 to 45 minutes with music portions lasting from 3 to 20 minutes.

CHAPTER FOUR

Variations in the Selection and Use of Music

The individual Bonny Method session is defined by the use of predesigned programs of classical music (Bruscia, 2002a). Group GIM is not defined by the sole use of classical music or predesigned programs; therefore, the use of other types of music and extemporaneous programming in group sessions does not constitute modification of the Bonny Method.

The most common modified approach to programming is spontaneous. Though not typically specified in the clinical literature, there are three types of spontaneous programming: moving from one program to another before the previous program is heard in its entirety; moving from piece to piece within a preselected group of related pieces; and moving from any piece to any other piece as needed. In addition, a new "music-centered" approach to programming in individual GIM has been designed for general purposes (Summer, 2009). Due to its recent inception, this approach to programming was not included in the survey. Any approaches to programming that do not involve the use of predesigned programs are considered modifications of the Bonny Method, as are any uses of nonclassical music.

Most Frequent Practices

The survey research was focused on individual practices and revealed that predesigned music programs were still being used often or always by most practitioners (89%), while spontaneous programming was used often or sometimes by many practitioners (62%). The three types of spontaneous programming were in use: 70% of those who practiced spontaneous programming moved from piece to piece as needed often or sometimes, 80% moved from piece to piece within a group of pieces often or sometimes, and 61% moved from one program to another often or sometimes. Classical music was still being used often or always when predesigning programs by 94% of practitioners and when programming extemporaneously, by 89%. Movie, world, and New Age music were used sometimes or less often by most practitioners (85%), and pop music was used rarely. In summary, extemporaneous programming and nonclassical music were in use, but much less often than the Bonny Method standards of predesigned programs and classical music.

A comparison of session length and music length with age and populations served indicated that some of them may vary in relation to each other. For example, practitioners who more frequently worked with adolescents also tended to more often use world music when designing programs and when programming extemporaneously, while they used classical music less often. Those who worked with well adults more often tended to more frequently program extemporaneously during a less-than-1½-hour session and to more frequently use classical music when designing programs. Practitioners who more frequently worked with normal neuroses tended to more often move from one program to another when programming extemporaneously and to more often use movie music when programming extemporaneously. Those who more frequently treated clients with anxiety and/or depression tended to more frequently use predesigned programs and to more frequently use classical music when programming extemporaneously, while they tended not to program extemporaneously during a less-than-1½-hour session. Practitioners who tended to work more often with psychological trauma tended less often to use classical music when designing programs. These findings are consistent with the literature that is covered in the next section.

Specific Practices

The clinical literature on GIM provides many insights into why and how the selection and uses of music are modified for individual sessions. The literature also provides insights into the selection and use of music in group sessions. The discussion of the literature in this chapter has been organized into four main groups of clientele:

psychiatric, physical illness, elderly, and children. Unless specified, references to music selections in this chapter represent single pieces or short programs of classical music predesigned by the authors.

Psychiatric

Classical music that is stable and supportive, mostly legato with moderate tempi, minimal dynamic variation and harmonic tension, few harmonic themes, and little development (e.g., Bach's *Air on a G String*; Pachelbel's *Canon in D*; Mozart's *Clarinet Concerto in F Major*, 2nd movement) has been recommended for early individual sessions (Ritchey Vaux, 1993; Summer, 1998) and for vulnerable clients with weak egos in individual and/or group inpatient treatment (Blake, 1994; Blake & Bishop, 1994; Goldberg, 1994; Moe, 2002; Moe, Rosen, & Raben, 2000). Goldberg (1994) has referred to the use of stable and supportive New Age music (e.g., works by Daniel Kobialka) as well for this population. Note that the use of nonclassical music represents an adaptation in terms of individual work, but not in terms of group work (Bruscia, 2002a). Stable and supportive classical music has also been used for the treatment of psychologically fragile clients in private settings (Clarkson, 1995; Summer & Chong, 2006; Wrangsjö, 1994). These authors use this type of music because it tends to help clients to maintain and work in shallow altered states of consciousness and inspires them to generate manageable amounts and types of imagery.

Other authors have reported using more evocative classical music that is also stable and supportive, while also encouraging imagery to develop (e.g., Debussy's *Prelude to the Afternoon of a Fawn*; Strauss's *A Hero's Life*). This stable yet evocative music has been used in subsequent sessions (Ritchey Vaux, 1993; Summer, 1998), as client ego strength increases (Clarkson, 1995; Summer & Chong, 2006), and for groups of clients in drug and alcohol recovery (Moe, 2011–2012; Murphy, 2008; Skaggs, 1997a). The use of specific types of classical music for these purposes does not constitute adaptation of the Bonny Method.

There is, however, a clear boundary in terms of the use of predesigned music programs. The BMGIM is defined by the use of predesigned programs each with "its own affective contour, sensitively timed to lead the traveler into a particular state of consciousness and/or emotional space, hold the traveler there, and then provide a pathway out or back" (Bruscia, 2002a, p. 56). The authors above who have written about uses of music with psychiatric patients and those below who write about uses of music with the physically ill, the elderly, and children and adolescents seem to have indicated that certain clients are unable to safely or effectively go on the types of inner journeys on which the GIM programs are designed to take a person. In lieu of the predesigned programs that have been created for GIM, these authors have selected single pieces of music or perhaps two or three short pieces of similar music. Whereas these selections may have been chosen and arranged prior to a given session, they are not equivalent to the predesigned programs that have become part of the standard GIM repertoire. Standard GIM programs are developed through an extended and rigorous process and are designed to be used with a range of clients. Therefore, shorter programs of stable and supportive classical music that are created in less time to address specific client needs represent adapted practice.

Specific recommendations for the selection and use of classical music have been made for traumatized clients. In choosing music for early sessions with traumatized clients, therapists were cautioned against selecting classical music that is rhythmically or harmonically transient, dissonant, dynamic, or otherwise evocative (Korlin, 2002). The use of less active music that is more consonant, with more predictable and consistent harmonic structures and with no dynamic surprises, can help to build trust and safety between the traumatized client and the music and between the therapist and the client while they are listening to the music (Hahna & Borling, 2003–2004; Moffitt & Hall, 2003–2004; Smith, 1996–1997). If the client tends to avoid emotion and intimate relationships, which is characteristic of clients with PTSD, classical music with these potentials should also be avoided in the beginning of GIM work (Korlin, 2002). For traumatized clients who are hypersensitive to any type of music or who feel threatened by it, therapists must exert great care in identifying classical music that will help clients to feel relaxed, comfortable, safe, and secure as they travel (Hahna & Borling, 2003–2004; Korlin, 2002).

In contrast, Korlin (2002) has found that clients with severe PTSD or who were traumatized at a young age may be distrustful of music that is consonant, structured, and predictable and feel more at home with music that matches their internal, insecure state, i.e., music that is dissonant, less structured, and less predictable. Moffitt and Hall (2003–2004) disagreed with Korlin's finding and noted that, in their particular case study, a client who had suffered extensive abuse in childhood and who had severe symptoms of PTSD, was immediately comforted and strengthened by consonant, structured, and predictable music. Regardless of which music works for a given client, use of this specially selected classical music over a series of sessions can help the client to gradually build ego strength and prepare for deeper work (Korlin, 2002). Korlin (2002) has also described the use of this music as a supportive presence while the client travels at a more shallow level and receives direct support from the therapist. To assess the client's ability to move into deeper work, Korlin (2002) recommends the use of classical music that varies dynamically but is otherwise stable (e.g., Beethoven's *Fifth Piano Concerto,* 2nd movement), as the dynamic swells may bring traumatic material to the surface.

For clients with Dissociative Identity Disorder (DID), formerly Multiple Personality Disorder (MPD), specific pieces of choral music may be preselected to facilitate a gathering of ego states. According to Pickett and Sonnen (1993), shifts from one personality to another can be abrupt and unexpected; these personality shifts may be triggered by psychosocial stress, elicited by verbal request, and also initiated by music. Once they are initiated and gathered together, choral music can allow the different egos to express themselves and to be heard simultaneously. Bringing different ego states to the surface and facilitating communication among them is an important goal for clients with DID.

As explained earlier, selecting classical music to make the expansion and exploration of consciousness more manageable does not represent an adaptation of the Bonny Method; however, it does represent adaptation when it does not include the use of predesigned GIM programs.

The practice of spontaneous programming has been specifically referred to by several authors. Summer (1988) and Summer and Chong (2006) have used spontaneous programming to respond to individual psychiatric clients in the moment during music imaging. These applications seem partially based on client need and partially based on the therapist's theoretical orientation (Summer, 1992, 1995, 1998, 2009), namely psychodynamic, which represents another type of modification that is covered in Chapter Five. Moffitt and Hall (2003–2004) have changed music programs and substituted pieces to accommodate a traumatized client who was extremely sensitive to sound. Smith (1996–1997) wrote about shifting to stronger music in the moment once her traumatized client connected to her anger "to sustain that emotion and facilitate the necessary catharsis" (p. 13).

Physical Illness

Goldberg, Hoss, and Chesna (1988) chose a mixture of structured non-GIM classical and New Age music to help a brain-damaged patient to contain her affect and anxiety and to structure her images and thoughts. To adjust to the needs of medical patients, Wigle-Justice and Kasayka (1999) recommended structured, repetitive, and nonambiguous GIM pieces and New Age selections to help patients maintain and/or deepen a given imagery focus. GIM music with slow tempi, consistent dynamics and rhythms, predictable diatonic harmonies, and legato phrasing has also been used to work with patients in end-of-life care who are often sensitive to noise and who do not have the energy to handle music with strong emotional content (Marr, 1998–1999). As described earlier in the psychiatric section, the use of specific types of music in lieu of predesigned GIM programs for the physically ill represents modification of the Bonny Method.

Elderly

Summer (1981) chose music from the standard GIM repertoire to match the mood of nursing home residents and help them to focus on inner awareness, to increase their self-esteem, and to spark their motivation. For open group sessions at a nursing home, Short (1992, 2007) used single pieces of supportive classical music and avoided selections from depth-oriented GIM programs. The music on these programs (e.g., Grieving, Death-Rebirth, Affect Release) is contraindicated for persons with limited insight and ego strength, poor cognitive skills, and severe physical illness and for those who are taking mind-altering medications and/or might be experiencing hallucinations and confusion.

Children and Adolescents

Wesley (2002) used single selections of New Age or classical music for individual sessions with three boys in a locked psychiatric unit. The boys, ages 6, 7, and 10, were given the opportunity to select a piece of music to match a starting image. Skaggs (1997b) used single pieces of classical music to provide a sense of safety, containment, and grounding for groups of juvenile sex offenders who were concurrently confronting their offense(s) as well as their own victimization. As an example of such music, she mentioned Vivaldi's *Guitar Concerto in D*, which is characterized by "74 pulses per minute, well within the range of the beat of a healthy heart at rest. The strong bass line throughout the movement gives a deep sense of support and predictability" (Skaggs, 1997b, p. 75).

Classical music selections have been used with groups of normal and disadvantaged children of ages 4–8 and 8–11 to introduce them to this type of music and to expose them to creative problem-solving via the altered state of consciousness during music listening (Summer, 1988). Roy (1996–1997) used single pieces of classical music with high school girls to reduce stress and to build self-esteem by exposing them to a deeper experience of inner feelings and concerns and to inner creativity. Powell (2007–2008) described the use of simple and consonant classical pieces with a clear beginning, middle, and end and slow tempi to help high-risk elementary school children to relax and gain self-insight.

General-Purpose

Summer (2009) has created a form of spontaneous music programming that involves the repetition of pieces of classical music during the music imaging phase of an individual GIM session. Summer explained that this *music-centered* approach to programming was not developed to accommodate the health needs of a specific client population. Instead, it was inspired by the needs of experienced GIM travelers, although she suggests that it may be useful with a range of clients.

In this approach to programming, the therapist extemporaneously chooses and links pieces of music based on the client's in-the-moment experience and repeats one or more of these pieces one or more times. The idea is to hold the client in one piece of music so that she or he can have a deeper, more intimate, and more immediate encounter with the music. Summer has identified three types of repetition: *music-oriented, transformation-oriented,* and *introjection-oriented*. Music-oriented repetition occurs at the beginning of a program to help the client have a more internalized experience of a given piece. The intention here is not to support the client's imagery but rather "to open or deepen the client's relational capacity toward the music" (p. 288). Transformation-oriented repetition occurs in the middle of a program. "Whereas introducing new musical material tends to bring change, repeated musical material may deepen and support the content of transformational imagery as it emerges" (p. 288). Introjection-oriented repetition occurs toward the end of a program when the client is having a transpersonal experience. The intention here is to use repeated listening to help the client internalize positive feelings, especially at a physical level. In addition, Summer suggests that using one piece of music and repeating it may be more effective for first-time travelers than using a program with varied pieces that would evoke many images, such as Bonny's "Explorations" program, which is commonly used for a client's first session (Bruscia, 1991, 2003). Summer's innovative approach to programming clearly represents a modification of the Bonny Method.

Summary

In summary, modified forms of programming and nonclassical music have been reported in the literature for use in individual sessions with psychiatric, physically ill, and child clients. Nonclassical music has been used to limit the expansion and exploration of consciousness for psychologically or physically fragile clients but more often specific types of classical music, typically consonant and structured music, are used to do so. Specific types of classical music are also chosen to match a client's inner state, which can be experienced as consonant or dissonant, structured or unstructured. Spontaneous programming has been used to respond to client need in the moment. A new "music-centered" approach to programming involves choosing music pieces to meet the clients' needs in the moment and repeating one or more of these pieces to limit the generation and exploration of imagery and to deepen the client's experience of the music.

Variations in group work include the use of structured classical music and nonclassical music to limit the expansion and exploration of consciousness for psychologically or physically fragile psychiatric, physically ill, and child clients.

Chapter Five

Variations in Verbal Dialogue and Guiding

The individual Bonny Method session is defined by a nondirective approach to verbal dialogue and guiding (Bruscia, 2002a). Any directive verbal or physical interventions during any part of the session and any music imaging that does not involve a steady verbal exchange between the client and therapist are modifications of the Bonny Method. In Group GIM, the travelers image alone without dialogue or intervention from the therapist; therefore, any intervention during the music imaging during a group session is considered a modification.

Both the survey and the clinical literature suggest that various types of verbal dialogue and guiding interventions in individual and group sessions are being used to accommodate a variety of client health concerns. A new "music-centered" approach to guiding in individual GIM has also been designed for general purposes (Summer, 2009). Due to its recent inception, this approach to programming was not included in the survey. Note that Summer's music-centered approach to guiding, which is considered a modification, is not to be confused with music-centered interventions that are a Bonny Method practice (Bruscia, 2002a). In addition, a variety of group session forms for general purposes that have been detailed in the literature are included in this chapter. These were not included in the survey, as their frequency of use was considered to be limited.

Most Frequent Practices

The survey research was focused on individual practices and revealed that Bonny Method practices were still being used often or always by most practitioners. Specifically, dialogue during the music imaging was being used often or always (89%), music-centered interventions often or always (80%), and physical interventions when requested by the client often or always (54%). In contrast, modified practices were used less: 78% of practitioners used directive interventions during the prelude and postlude sometimes or less often. Theoretical interpretation during the prelude and/or postlude was used sometimes or less often by 80% of practitioners. In general, most practitioners (88%) used directive guiding techniques sometimes or less often. The following modified practices were used sometimes or less often by most practitioners: introducing an image during the music experience (92%), physical interventions when the need is perceived by the therapist (79%), having the client sit in an upright position during the music imaging (97%), and having the client image with eyes open (99%).

The survey revealed that GIM fellows who practice within the United States use physical interventions when they perceive that the client needs them more frequently than those who practice outside the United States. This may be explained by cultural differences, although a wide variety of cultures was included in the "outside the United States" category. Perhaps physical touch is more accepted in U.S. culture than it is in the cultures of the other countries as a whole. Therapists from different cultures may be trained differently about the use of physical touch, and clients in different cultures may have different needs and expectations about physical touch within the context of therapy.

A comparison of types of verbal dialogue and guiding interventions with age and populations served indicated that some of them may vary in relation to each other. For example, the more often practitioners worked with adults, the more often they used music-centered interventions and the more often they used physical interventions when requested by the client. This finding reflects two Bonny Method practices that have traditionally been used with adults. The more frequently practitioners worked with psychosis, the more frequently they tended to introduce an image during the music experience. This is consistent with the literature on psychosis that is covered in the next section. Conversely, the more often practitioners worked with substance abuse/addiction and/or adolescents, the less often they tended to use starting images. There is no mention in the literature of not using starting images with these populations. In addition, the more often practitioners worked with adolescents, the less often they used verbal dialogue during the music imaging or physical interventions when requested by the client. Most of the reported work with adolescents is within unguided group sessions; it also seems instinctive to avoid physical intervention with this population. Practitioners who worked with anxiety and/or depression more often tended to use physical interventions when requested by the client less often, and those who more often worked with terminal illness tended to use music-centered interventions less frequently. There is no support for these findings in the literature.

Specific Practices

The clinical literature on GIM provides many insights into why and how verbal dialogues and guiding interventions are modified in individual and in group sessions. The discussion of the literature in this chapter has been organized into three main groups of clientele: psychiatric, physical illness, and children. Note that any use of GIM with groups for therapeutic purposes is a modification of Group GIM; therefore, the interventions used to facilitate this work are detailed in this section. All other modifications are specifically referred to below.

Psychiatric

Goldberg (1994), Summer (1988), and Summer and Chong (2006) have directed verbal discussion during the prelude of individual sessions for psychiatric clients with compromised ego functioning. It seems that this was done for two reasons: to set clear boundaries for GIM work and to limit the focus to acute symptoms. To prepare clients for the music, these same authors provided simple inductions and starting images focused on specific symptoms. Applying Bruscia's (2002a) distinctions here, even if a therapist maintains a nondirective approach to guiding during the music imaging, the use of directive or nondirective interventions that are formulated from other than a humanistic or transpersonal orientation during any other part of the session is an adaptation of the Bonny Method. Using GIM to focus on acute symptoms seems to raise the need for another distinction. Using directive interventions to help make the expansion and exploration of consciousness through free and spontaneous music imaging more manageable to a patient in acute psychiatric care is not the same as doing so in order to target behavioral goals (e.g., to reduce anxiety, to decrease physical tension, to develop coping skills, etc.). The former seems to constitute the use of behavioral techniques within a humanistic approach, whereas the latter constitutes a behavioral orientation to GIM work. In the clinical literature, it is often unclear which theoretical orientation was being used by an author during different phases of a session. When authors do refer to theoretical orientations, they often do so without tying them to specific interventions. Further survey data and literature on theoretical orientations to GIM will be covered in Chapter Six. Goldberg (1994), Summer (1988), and Summer and Chong (2006) also used directive guiding during the music imaging to help patients form defensive maneuvers and generate positive images (e.g., "Find a safe place," "Move away from her," "Protect yourself," etc.). Any directive guiding during the music imaging is a modification of the Bonny Method (Bruscia, 2002a).

In her limited work with individual hospitalized patients with severe personality disorder, Bonny (2002g) described the need to employ directive guiding, to provide immediate reinforcement and constant contact. Due to patients' abrupt mood changes and abreactions, she noted, guiding these patients required so much focus and energy that she was unable to maintain a transcript. Bonny also had a hospital aide, who would later be available in the unit, attend the GIM session. Note that the use of directive guiding by Bonny is not a defining feature of the Bonny Method because Bruscia's (2002a) definitions are based on work that she developed over a period of time through work with a range of clients.

Other specific variations and modifications for the use of GIM with traumatized clients have appeared in the literature. These include dialogues with the client during the induction to ensure that he or she is responding positively and achieving relaxation (Hahna & Borling, 2003–2004) and specifically designed and repeatedly used inductions (Moffitt & Hall, 2003–2004) to create a reliable and consistent sense of safety. Moffit and Hall (2003–2004) also described having the client image a color that may bring feelings of nurturance. When protective relationships from the client's past are identified, they can serve as the focus in preparation for the music (Korlin, 2002). These variations constitute adaptations only if they were formulated from other than a humanistic or transpersonal orientation which was not specified by the authors. Variations in the use of inductions were not included in the survey.

Hahna and Borling (2003–2004) reported that directive guiding and physical interventions are commonly used by therapists during the music imaging with traumatized clients. When transitioning clients from Music Breathing (MB), a technique that includes therapist-directed breathing exercises and music listening, to BMGIM, Korlin (2007–2008) uses both directive MB interventions and nondirective GIM guiding techniques.

Along with the music choices for clients with Dissociative Identity Disorder, the guide can dialogue with the client's different ego states during the music to bring them to the surface and to facilitate communication among them (Pickett & Sonnen, 1993). An essential part of this process is the fostering of leadership traits in one of the more responsible personalities, if this has not already happened naturally. This executive ego "can promote purpose, identity, and healing in the overall system, and can also function as a cotherapist" (Pickett & Sonnen, 1993, p. 60). It is also useful for the various ego states to have a space in the imagery that is neutral, a gathering space that feels safe and comfortable to each of them. Pickett and Sonnen (1993) have recommended ending GIM sessions with an imagery exercise referred to as an ecology check. In it, the therapist guides the client to imagine the meeting place and invites all of the ego states to gather together. The therapist then checks in with each and invites them to share their reaction(s) to the session, especially with each other. The goal is to "make sure that any changes or revealed traumata don't inadvertently challenge, corner, or threaten some aspect of the system's functioning" (Pickett & Sonnen, 1993, p. 69). It seems that GIM for clients with DID involves a significant amount of directive guiding, regardless of whether a given ego state is at the surface when the guide intervenes.

In her GIM work with a nonverbal autistic man, Clarkson (1995) was unable to guide the client during the music imaging. Whereas her client, Jerry, was unable to speak, he was high-functioning and could understand verbal communication. To communicate with him during preludes and postludes, Clarkson used a technique known as *facilitated communication*. This involved her supporting Jerry's left elbow as he typed his thoughts and responses into a laptop computer. When using this technique, the preludes were otherwise typical. In synch with the shorter session structure and the client's emotional and cognitive limitations, Clarkson provided inductions that were brief and simplified (e.g., deep breaths). During the music, Clarkson carefully observed her client's nonverbal responses to the music. Postludes involved Jerry drawing a mandala immediately after the music and then, with the assistance of the therapist, typing out and processing his music imaging experience. The absence of dialogue during the music in individual sessions is a modification of the Bonny Method (Bruscia, 2002a). The other aspects of Clarkson's work referred to above do not constitute modifications as per Bruscia (2002a) unless they were formulated from within other than a humanistic or transpersonal orientation which was not specified by the author.

For group sessions in inpatient psychiatry that include more fragile patients, the therapist may have them remain seated during the entire session (Goldberg, 1994) and have them keep their eyes open for the music imaging (Blake & Bishop, 1994). In GIM, the optimal position for music imaging is lying down with eyes closed (Bonny, 2002g), yet spontaneous imaging in an expanded state of consciousness is possible while sitting upright and with eyes open. In terms of adaptation to the Bonny Method, having patients travel in these ways falls into the same category as the uses of structured classical music. In both cases, the therapist is working to help clients have a manageable experience of expanding and exploring consciousness. If, however, these practices were used to help clients listen in an ordinary or relaxed state of consciousness the work would be considered an adaptation. In addition, any group sessions that are formulated with therapeutic goals for the clients constitute adaptations.

These GIM sessions for groups of hospitalized psychiatric patients may include directed imagery that is open-ended (e.g., "Allow an image to form that represents yourself ... take notice of the various features ..."), theme-oriented (e.g., "Many of you are preparing for discharge ... imagine yourself leaving the facility, notice how you feel ...") (Goldberg, 1994), or scene-oriented (e.g., a visit to a garden, a sailing trip, exploring a house) (Moe, Roesen, & Raben, 2000). Although spontaneous imaging is not discouraged, directed imagery may be provided for part (Moe, Roesen, & Raben, 2000), for most (Goldberg, 1994), or for the entire duration of the music (Moe, Roesen, & Raben, 2000). This may be done to help patients structure their inner experiences, to limit the development of potentially threatening imagery, and to decrease their chance of being overwhelmed. These practices seem to represent types of contained spontaneous imaging, which is an adaptation of the Bonny Method, although some seem to closely resemble directed music imaging, which is a music therapy technique (Bruscia, 2002a). To meet the same aims described above during nondirected travel, an induction and starting image that are highly specific may be followed by music imaging that is supported by writing, drawing, or movement (Blake & Bishop, 1994). Goldberg (1994) had patients begin writing their images down as soon as the directed imagery concluded yet while the music was still playing. These authors referred to this work as GIM; however, having clients write, draw, or move during music imaging seems to represent projective listening, which is a music therapy technique (Bruscia, 2002a).

Physical Illness

Individual sessions for medically fragile patients typically begin with verbal discussion to assess their physical and mental state and their readiness for inner work (Wigle-Justice & Kasayka, 1999). Following this, a gentle induction with a focus on safety, inner strength, and healing that is directly or indirectly related to the patient's symptoms may be used. Within this structure, the therapist can then guide the patient in imaging freely and spontaneously with the music and thereby accessing inner resources. Patients who cannot lie down comfortably due to certain medical procedures or following major surgery may remain seated during individual sessions (Short, 1999). During the postlude, the therapist can provide verbal reinforcement to help the patient bond in waking consciousness with aspects of the experience that can help them to cope with their illness (Wigle-Justice & Kasayka, 1999). After the music, the therapist can have the patient draw in order to concretize the experience and create a tangible link to valuable resources. As explained earlier in regard to psychiatric patients, the interventions referred to above would constitute adaptation of the BMGIM only if they were formulated from within other than a humanistic or transpersonal orientation. Wigle-Justice and Kasayka (1999) specifically refer to a transpersonal approach to work in medical care; Short (1999) did not specify. Following the same precepts, GIM can also be used with groups of fragile medical patients. The content of the relaxation, focus, and music can be similar to that used with individuals, but all patients may sit rather than lie down for the experience. Verbal dialogue and drawings can be used to process the experience while patients gain social support from each other and learn a range of coping options by hearing the experiences of others. In general, the interventions described above and below in work with the physically ill represent adaptations in terms of the use of GIM with groups for therapeutic purposes.

Goldberg, Hoss, and Chesna (1988) discussed how, in a specific case, the therapist's use of concrete stimuli (e.g., a picture on the wall) and support of kinesthetic imaging (e.g., physical movement, making sounds) helped a brain damaged patient to fully engage in music imaging during individual sessions. For most of the sessions, the therapist had the patient, who was already in an altered state of consciousness due to her injury, image with her eyes open and helped her to maintain more concrete (e.g., a favorite vacation spot) and less fantasy-oriented experiences. To help alleviate the client's anxiety, the therapist suggested that she imagine the therapist accompanying her within her travel. The therapist did not engage the client in verbal processing of her images due to the client's lack of short-term memory. These practices were referred to as GIM by the authors, but it seems that there was a mixture of projective listening and directed music imaging (music therapy), along with contained spontaneous imaging (GIM). The use of directive guiding makes these practices an adaptation of the Bonny Method.

When guiding an individual session with the terminally ill, it is important to follow the patients' lead and allow them to move out of difficult images if they wish and to guide them toward positive aspects of the music imaging experience (Marr, 1998–1999). At the request of one terminally ill patient, there was no dialogue during the music, and images were reported and processed afterward (Marr, 1998–1999). The use of directive guiding and the absence of guiding during music imaging in individual sessions both represent modifications of the Bonny Method.

Elderly

For group sessions with nursing home residents, Summer (1981) has started with a five-minute progressive relaxation followed by an image of travel (e.g., taking a trip outside of the home) or memory (e.g., pleasant family event). To decrease the possibility of residents falling asleep, Summer (1981) has recommended suggesting that the relaxation exercise and the music will stimulate and energize. When no facilities were available to transfer elderly disabled clients to a more comfortable position, Short (1992) encouraged them to become comfortable in their wheelchairs. Short (2007) has started sessions with gentle physical exercise to music and has initiated discussion of relaxing places and activities. Due to the physical discomfort of her clients and their lack of mobility, Short (1992) avoided progressive muscle relaxations. To establish a similar focus and beginning state of consciousness for all group members, Short (1992) presented very specific and succinct starting images, some of which she solicited spontaneously from the residents. Short (2007) has encouraged residents to choose a real or imaginary relaxing place on which to focus during the music imaging. In cases where group discussion was not forthcoming, popular music was used to gradually bring the residents back to an alert state (Short, 2007). Sessions led by Short (2007) have also concluded with morning tea, during which she observed and interacted with the residents individually and offered assistance to those with ongoing emotional reactions or who had not fully returned from the altered state of consciousness. In general, these interventions represent adaptations in terms of the use of GIM with groups for therapeutic purposes. The use of directive interventions and the use of nonclassical music are also adaptations of the Bonny Method.

Children and Adolescents

During individual sessions in a locked psychiatric unit, Wesley (2002) had the children start sessions by singing a favorite song. She then provided a breathing relaxation with music and had the child choose from a list of starting imagery scenes (e.g., sitting by a small pond, looking out from a mountaintop, the sun on a cocooned caterpillar). Each child also chose a colored scarf as an accompanying prop (e.g., a raft, a magic carpet, a cocoon). Wesley did not specify whether sessions were guided or unguided. Processing included drawing and discussion. Her goals for the children seemed humanistic, namely to heighten awareness and provide a fresh sense of reality, and she found that the sessions helped the boys to gain coping skills for daily living. Bruscia (2002a) does not refer to the use of active music-making before or after music imaging; however, this variation in practice was covered in the survey. In addition, it does seem that Wesley (2002) used some directive interventions to help the patients have a manageable experience.

For groups of juvenile sex offenders, Skaggs (1997b) instructed the boys to image a place where they felt safe, and she allowed them to decide whether to close their eyes. Skaggs found that Group GIM helped these boys to find an inner place of safety, which was a healthy preparation for dealing with their own victimization. Drawing was used to process these experiences, and the therapist encouraged them to use their internal safe places to help them manage emotions and behaviors in times of stress.

In a group format, Summer (1988) has described having disadvantaged and normal children of ages 4–8 each draw an animal to serve as the focus for music imaging. The children were asked to draw again after the music to process. With groups of mostly high-risk children in the 3rd through 8th grades, Powell (2007–2008) has used verbal discussion to briefly describe the GIM process and to set expectations of mutual respect, quiet, and personal space boundaries. She used a brief breathing induction and a specific starting focus based on a theme or topic identified during the discussion (e.g., finding a safe place, making friends, focusing attention). For the music imaging, Powell has had the children put their heads down on their desks and, when space was available, to lie down on mats or rugs. During the music, she moved around the room to observe and to offer support and encouragement. Afterward, the children are invited to process the experience by writing, drawing, or sharing verbally.

Using Group GIM in a high school classroom setting, Roy (1996–1997) has provided students with an overview of visualization and relaxation techniques, symbolism, theories of color and shape, and the processing of dreams. At the beginning of each session, Roy has instructed the girls either to write about or to openly discuss their current feelings. They then chose to either put their heads down on their desks or lie down on the floor. A brief induction was provided followed by the music imaging. After the music, the girls were given the option of sharing their experience with others, but all were required to process their experience through writing or drawing a mandala.

The various interventions listed above with children and adolescents represent only adaptations of Group GIM in terms of group sessions for therapeutic purposes.

General-Purpose

Another music-centered modification created by Summer (2009) involves guiding the client toward the music. Here the therapist directs the client toward his or her experience of the music while other aspects of the client's imagery experience are tied to the music or deemphasized. Summer identified four types of music-centered guiding interventions: listening to the music (e.g., "Listen more deeply to the music"), describing the music (e.g., "What do you notice about the music?"), deferring to the music (e.g., "What does the music say?"), and tying the imagery to the music (e.g., "Is your mother hearing the music?"). Note that these interventions are part of the Bonny Method, but using them exclusively is not. This approach also seems to involve the use of directive guiding. The goal of music-centered guiding is to help the client to have a more intimate relationship with the music and for the music to serve as the client's primary therapist. Interestingly, Summer reports that while this type of guiding helps to bring the client closer to the music, it simultaneously creates a more intimate feeling between the client and the therapist and between the therapist and the music.

Additional types of Group GIM that can be used for general purposes have been described by Bruscia (2002a). These types of group music imaging experiences (summarized below) represent innovations that are underreported in the GIM literature. Specific types of sessions are not included in the survey, but the adaptations that they contain in terms of dialogue (with the therapist or other clients) or in terms of guiding (directive or nondirective) during group sessions are represented.

Contained spontaneous imaging. The guide presents the group with an image and periodically directs them to explore different locations or aspects of it. As they explore each location or aspect, the guide serves as a supportive presence but does not intervene while each client images freely and spontaneously.

Group reimaging (unguided). The guide prepares the group to enter the previous image or dream of one of the group members. The guide serves as a supportive presence while each member images freely and spontaneously within the image or dream to a short excerpt of the same music that was associated with the original experience.

Group reimaging (guided). After one member of the group describes an important image or dream and chooses members of the group to enter it with him/her, the guide prepares the group. During the travel, the guide uses standard nondirective guiding to engage the participants in an interactive and solution-oriented dialogue.

Progressive group imaging. The guide instructs the group members that they will each verbally contribute to an evolving image or story during the music. After providing a relaxation induction and perhaps a starting image, the guiding is limited. The guide may ensure that each member contributes and that they contribute in turn and may guide them in filling out or completing the image or story and bringing the experience to a close.

Group go-rounds on individual. The guide instructs the group members that one at a time they will each become the focus of the music imaging. After an image or story involving the member of focus is determined, the guide assists one of the other group members in traveling to it with or without guidance during the music and without interference from the member of focus. The guide then assists another group member, then the next, and so on.

Individual go-rounds on group. The guide instructs the group that one member will image something about each of them. The guide assists the group member in imagining being a character (e.g., an animal) or taking on some role (e.g., conscience of the group) and then, one at a time, making each other group member the focus of his/her travel. This may or may not develop into a dialogue between the two members, and the guide may or may not guide them.

Group co-imaging (1). All group members are guided in cocreating an imagery experience. The guide provides a starting image, placing each member into the scene and then inviting them to interact. Using standard nondirective techniques, the guide guides each of them and the entire group as the image evolves.

Group co-imaging (2). All of the group members are guided in cocreating an imagery experience. The guide provides the group with a starting image and invites them to image on their own and verbally relate their individual experiences to the group when they feel moved to do so. Gradually, with the guide guiding them, their separate journeys become a shared experience.

Summary

In summary, modified approaches to verbal dialogue and guiding have been reported in the literature for use in individual and sessions with psychiatric, physically ill, and child clients. Directed verbal discussion has been used during the prelude, induction, and postlude to limit the expansion and exploration of consciousness and to focus on acute symptoms or positive resources. Live music-making and drawing have also been used during the prelude and postlude. Directive guiding has been used to provide clients with immediate contact and reinforcement, to guide them toward positive experiences, and to induce ego states and facilitate communication among them. Music imaging portions have also been facilitated without verbal dialogue between client and therapist for clients with limited communication or at the client's request. Music imaging has also been guided with clients sitting up and in some cases with eyes open to accommodate physical or cognitive limitations. Music-centered guiding involves the therapist directing the client's focus toward the music while minimizing the imagery focus.

Verbal dialogue and guiding have also been reported for use in group sessions with psychiatric, physically ill, elderly, child, and adolescent clients. The use of any verbal dialogue or guiding and/or the use of sessions used for therapeutic purposes represent modifications to Group GIM. Specific techniques are applied to work with groups for the same purposes summarized above for individual sessions. Additional types of Group GIM for general use have been described, namely, contained spontaneous imaging, group re-imaging (unguided), group re-imaging (guided), progressive group imaging, group go-rounds on individual, and two forms of group co-imaging. These represent modifications in terms of the use of verbal dialogue and guiding during group sessions.

Chapter Six

Variations in Theoretical Orientation

The individual and group forms of the Bonny Method are defined by the use of a humanistic/existential or transpersonal/spiritual orientation (Bruscia, 2002a). As indicated in Chapter Two, variances in theoretical orientation constitute modifications to the Bonny method.

Most Frequent Practices

The survey research was focused on individual practices. Seven theoretical orientations were included in the survey: humanistic/existential; psychodynamic; transpersonal/spiritual; Jungian; bioenergetic, somatic, and/or chakra; cognitive/behavioral; and Gestalt. An "other" option was also offered that allowed practitioners to type in an orientation not on the list. Practitioners were asked to choose their primary (only one) theoretical orientation to practice; therefore, what follows are the percentages of practitioners who chose that orientation, not how frequently they used it. Practitioners chose humanistic/existential (30%), followed by psychodynamic (22%), transpersonal/spiritual (19%), and Jungian (13%). Few indicated bioenergetic, somatic, and/or chakra (1%) or cognitive/behavioral (1%), and no practitioners indicated Gestalt as their primary theoretical orientation. The remaining 14% indicated an "other" orientation. These include: eclectic, integrative psychotherapy, feminist, and resource-oriented. Note that the psychodynamic and Jungian orientations were being used more frequently than the modified practices covered in previous chapters and that the gap between them and the Bonny Method orientations is not as wide.

Practitioners were also asked how frequently they use each of the seven theoretical orientations when formulating interventions during the prelude and postlude and during the music imaging. Most practitioners indicated using a Bonny Method orientation sometimes or more often during the prelude and postlude:

humanistic/existential (91%) and transpersonal/spiritual (88%). Two modified orientations were used often or sometimes during the prelude and postlude by most practitioners: psychodynamic (80%) and Jungian (77%). Here again, the gap between the use of Bonny Method orientations and psychodynamic and Jungian orientations during the prelude and postlude is not great. Only 52% of practitioners indicated using a Gestalt orientation often or sometimes during the prelude and postlude. Most sometimes or less often used a bioenergetic, somatic, and/or chakra orientation (89%) and/or a cognitive/behavioral orientation (89%). Most practitioners indicated using a Bonny Method orientation sometimes or more often during the music imaging: humanistic/existential (91%) and transpersonal/spiritual (91%). Three modified orientations were used often or sometimes during the music imaging by most practitioners: Jungian (76%), psychodynamic (71%), and bioenergetic, somatic, and/or chakra (62%). Again, in relation to the use of Bonny Method orientations, the use of these modified orientations during the music imaging is considerable. The remaining two orientations were used sometimes or less often during the music imaging by most practitioners: Gestalt (82%) and cognitive/behavioral (98%).

 A comparison of theoretical orientations used with age and populations served indicates that some of them may vary in relation to each other. Whereas the following findings do not contradict the literature, no direct support for them was found. Those who worked more frequently with older adults tended to more often use a transpersonal or spiritual orientation during the prelude and postlude. Practitioners who treated substance abuse/addiction more often tended to more often use a Gestalt orientation during the prelude and postlude. Conversely, those who worked with anxiety and/or depression more frequently tended less often to use a bioenergetic, somatic, and/or chakra orientation during the prelude and postlude and to less often use a psychodynamic orientation during the music. Practitioners who more frequently worked with cancer patients tended to less often use a Gestalt orientation during the prelude, postlude, and music imaging.

Specific Practices

Two orientations are found in the GIM literature: psychodynamic and Jungian. Whereas these orientations and their application to GIM have been described in detail, the literature does not indicate why a humanistic or transpersonal orientation would require modification. In addition, it is not clear that theoretical orientations are being used to accommodate health concerns; they may have more to do with therapist preference. Moreover, modifications of this type are not, for the most part, overtly evident in changes to the length of the session or music, the selection and use of music, or the therapist's interventions. When a therapist adopts a particular theoretical orientation, what changes is how the therapist views the client's entire process; this influences the therapist's stance in relation to the client as well as every decision that the therapist makes.

Psychodynamic

The two primary aims of psychodynamically oriented therapy are:

> (1) to bring into the client's conscious experience material from the past that had been repressed and kept in the unconscious through defenses and resistances and that exerts adverse psychological effects on the present and (2) to work through that material by using transference and countertransference to engage the client in corrective emotional experience (Bruscia, 1998b, p. 14).

In GIM, the first aim is achieved through the music imaging and is consistent with the Bonny Method. The second aim represents one way to understand modifications in this category, specifically, how the therapist configures the transference objects that are available to a client in a GIM session. Transference objects include the therapist, the music, and the client's images (Bruscia, 2002b). In addition, the therapist can be configured as a therapeutic ally rather than a transference object. The literature suggests that how the therapist understands, configures, and facilitates these dynamics, including the ones in which he or she consciously participates and the extent to which he or she manages countertransference reactions, determines how specifically the therapist is modifying BMGIM to fit within a psychodynamic orientation.

Summer (1998) suggests that in GIM the client's transferences exist on a continuum with the therapist on one end, the music on the other, and a split transference in the middle. Operating from this configuration, the therapist has the option of guiding the client's transferences away from the therapist and toward the music (Summer, 1998). For the client's first listening experience, Summer (1992, 1995, 1998, 2009) recommends music with an exposition that will match the client's internal state. This serves to hold the client while she or he merges with the music. Summer (1998) argues that the client's transference to the music is of greater importance than the client's transference to the therapist. She compares the relationship between the music and a client to the relationship between a mother and her newborn child. The music can provide for the client an experience of being held, understood, and nurtured, and Summer believes that it is the therapist's role to help the client to connect with the music in this way from the start. By developing a direct and pure transference with the music, the client can have what object relations theorist David Winnicott called a "good enough" nurturing experience (Summer, 1998). Following Winnicott's theory, Summer suggests that the therapist choose music that initially helps the client to have a *me* experience in relation to the music and then gradually expose the client to *not me* experiences as the music experience unfolds, as well as in subsequent sessions. *Not me* experiences are offered to child and client alike to "expand his abilities, behaviors, and feelings—expand his sense of being in the world" (Summer, 1992, p. 47). In the case examples that she provides, Summer (1998, 2009) uses shortened programs that consist of one to five classical pieces. Following the first selection, subsequent pieces are chosen spontaneously that follow the *me* experiences to match the immediate needs of the client. In fostering the pure music transference, the therapist configures the dynamics of a GIM session as dyadic: client–music.

Another type of dyadic configuration occurs when the therapist uses the music as an extension of or expression of him- or herself or as the therapist's vehicle within which the client travels (Izenberg-Grzeda, 1998). Here the therapist and music are one, and the dyadic configuration is client–therapist. In contrast to the pure music transference, the music as an extension of the therapist "promotes client resistance to awareness of the transference with the music, as well as resistance to involvement in the transference with the music" (Bruscia, 2002b, p. 239). A second form of client–therapist dyad occurs when the music is configured as the therapist's gift to the client (Izenberg-Grzeda, 1998). This stance by the therapist may in effect discourage the client from engaging in negative feelings toward the music or toward the therapist who has offered her or him a gift of music (Bruscia, 2002b; Izenberg-Grzeda, 1998).

When the therapist decides to utilize the split transference or to use the music as a cotherapist, the transference configuration is triadic: client–therapist–music (Bruscia, 2002b). Izenberg-Grzeda (1998) states that by using the music in this way, the therapist may help the client to relate to the therapist as a therapeutic ally rather than a transference object. Alternately, when the therapist is in whole or in part the object of the client's transference, the therapist can become many figures and manage many dynamics, both positive and negative, from the client's past (Bruscia, 1995). Clarkson and Geller (1996) suggest that when using the music as a cotherapist, the music can absorb some of the client's transference to the therapist. In other words, "the client and therapist can easily shift the more shadowy aspects of their relationship away from the therapist transference toward the music transference" (Bruscia, 2002b, p. 239). This implies that the client–therapist–music configuration depends largely on the extent of the therapist's generosity and flexibility (Bruscia, 1998c, 2000) in making him or herself available to the client as a transference object. Note that in each configuration of client transferences (client–music; client–therapist; client–therapist–music), there are implications for the therapist's countertransference reactions.

In addition to the therapist and the music, the characters or objects that clients create in their imagery can also be the foci of client transferences (Bruscia, 2002b). The therapist can view client images in three ways: as manifestations of the client's transferences to the music (Summer, 1998), as manifestations of the client's transferences to the therapist (Bruscia, 2002b; Pelliteri, 1998), or as introjects (manifestations of figures and dynamics from the client's past that she or he has incorporated into the self) (Bruscia, 2002b; Izenberg-Grzeda, 1998). Here again, each configuration has implications for the therapist's awareness of his or her countertransference.

In summary, there are at least four transference objects that are available to a client in a GIM session: therapist, music, imagery, and self (introjects). The client can also relate to the therapist's authentic self as therapist and ally in his or her treatment. Viewing these as a whole, Bruscia (2002b) offers:

> Moreover, in all likelihood, given the tendency of the unconscious to equate these objects and to replicate the past repeatedly but with endless variation, transferences toward multiple objects may not occur independently or without relation to one another. Instead, clients in BMGIM may develop an interdependent transference configuration directed toward two, three, or four objects, with each object implicated to a varying degree and with one in the foreground and the other in various background positions. When this is the case, a transference toward any one object cannot be completely understood without acknowledging transferences that may also be directed toward other objects at hand within the BMGIM process (p. 237).

Therefore, how the therapist understands and configures these dynamics, as well as the extent to which the therapist takes responsibility for the concomitant countertransference reactions, forms a basis for therapeutic decision-making and determines the extent and nature of modification to the Bonny Method.

Jungian

Several authors have described a Jungian approach to GIM (Brooks, 2000; Clark, 1991; Clarkson & Geller, 1996; Short, 1996–1997; Tasney, 1993; Ward, 2002; Warja, 1994; Wesley, 1998–1999). A Jungian approach to GIM includes fundamental psychodynamic concepts such as resistance, projection, and transference, but in the foreground are concepts originated by psychologist Carl Jung. Ward (2002) presents an overview of the concepts and constructs that are fundamental to a Jungian approach to therapy. The concept of opposites is present throughout Jung's theory, and the client's overall process is viewed as a journey toward individuation. Each client manifests to a greater or lesser degree certain opposite *psychological attitudes* (introversion and extroversion) and *psychological functions*, the rational (thinking and feeling), as well as the nonrational (intuition and sensation). Other poles are represented by the principles of *masculine* and *feminine* that transcend gender and are found in both men and women. Jung referred to the masculine in the female as her *animus*, and the feminine in the male as his *anima*; the integration of these is an important aspect of the client's process, and individuation is in part defined by achieving a balance between masculine and feminine (Brooks, 2000). A unique combination of these attitudes, functions, and principles is present in the client's *persona* (the mask one shows the world) and the client's *shadow* (the opposite of the mask; the unacceptable parts, whether positive or negative). As Ward points out, characters that embody the mask (idealized) and shadow (flawed) identities are universally present in fairy tales and legends. Jung used the terms *collective unconscious* and *archetypes* to represent and explain the universal appeal of these myths. "Our psychic heritage is reflected in the collective unconscious … which is the repository of all humankind's psychic heritage and possibilities" (Ward, 2002, p. 217).

A Jungian therapist may view the client's entire process as the unique manifestation of a single universal myth or a unique combination of myths. The characters that a client encounters internally or externally along his or her mythical journey toward individuation can be viewed as archetypal figures that are there sometimes to help, sometimes to challenge and thwart, and hopefully to ultimately be a source of greater self-knowing. This self-knowing can be understood in terms of the client's relationship between the *ego* and the *Self*. Whereas the ego represents the client's sense of identity, the Self is identity of a higher order, that which is present from birth to death, "the a priori inner determinant of our lives" (Ward, 2002, p. 218). A unifying concept is that of *complexes;* these are client responses that seem out of proportion or out of time with characters or events. "At the core of every complex are both a personal experience and an archetype related to it" (Ward, 2002, p. 218); the process of individuation brings these to the surface and requires acceptance and integration of them.

Therapists who take a Jungian approach to GIM listen for the manifestation of these various constructs in the clients' behaviors, in their descriptions of personal struggles and metaphors, in their drawings, in the ways they relate to the therapist and to different types of music, and certainly in the manifestation of the Jungian constructs within their imagery experiences (Brooks, 2000; Clark, 1991; Clarkson & Geller, 1996; Short, 1996–1997; Tasney, 1993; Ward, 2002; Warja, 1994; Wesley, 1998–1999). The therapist may also consider these constructs in relation to the potentials of specific inductions, starting images, and specific pieces of music or entire music programs (Ward, 2002) and, perhaps, when helping the client to interpret his or her experiences (Short, 1996–1997; Ward, 2002).

Summary

In summary, psychodynamic and Jungian theoretical orientations in individual sessions have been reported in the literature. Any use of an orientation other than humanistic or transpersonal constitutes a modification. When a therapist adopts a particular theoretical orientation, it colors every decision and action that is made on behalf of the client.

Chapter Seven

GIM Combined with Other Techniques and Methods

This chapter includes literature on the combination of GIM with another method or an involved technique. Each includes elements of the Bonny Method and/or modifications. These specific types of sessions were not included in the survey, but the adaptations they contain were represented and the findings included in previous chapters of this book.

Specific Practices

Directed Imagery and Music

Directed Imagery and Music (DIM) involves the combination of a facilitated recalling and re-experiencing of traumatic memories (Johnson, 1987) with GIM (Blake, 1994). In DIM, the prelude begins one week prior to the music imaging session. The client and the therapist meet and choose a single traumatic situation on which to focus. The client then verbally describes the event in as much detail as possible. One week later, the client describes the event again, along with any associated feelings. The therapist helps the client to relax and then orients him imaginatively to the time and place where the traumatic experience began. The client then describes the traumatic experience again and allows it to unfold accompanied by the music.

Music for DIM is chosen to accompany the client's inner experience, to reflect and anticipate the underlying emotion(s) leading up to and through the climax of the trauma, and to allow for reflection and closure. The length of the music experience depends on the length of the memory, often three to four pieces; however, additional pieces are made available for those who have deeper experiences. New Age music may be used for the reflection and closure portion of the music experience, as it can allow the client to more fully move out of intense emotion. As the client's experience unfolds through the music, the therapist employs standard nondirective guiding techniques. The goal of the music imaging is to provide opportunities for an integration and release of emotions and for reflection and closure. Blake (1994) designed DIM while working with combat veterans of the Vietnam War who were enrolled in an intensive 16-week inpatient PTSD program. The focus of the work was combat-related trauma. No other applications of DIM are found in the literature. Modifications to the Bonny Method here include a shortened music listening portion, the lack of predesigned GIM programs, and the use of New Age music (Bruscia, 2002a). In addition, the focus on a single traumatic memory resembles re-imaging, and like re-imaging, this is a type of contained spontaneous imaging.

Neurolinguistic Programming

Pickett and Sonnen (1993) describe the use of a neurolinguistic programming technique know as reframing (Grinder & Bandler, 1981) in conjunction with the Bonny Method for a client with Dissociative Identity Disorder (DID). During the prelude or the induction, the therapist establishes contact with the client's internal abuser and invites her or him to surface during the music experience and to engage in dialogue. The therapist assures the abuser that no attempt will be made to harm, reject, or get rid of him or her. The concept is that this part of the client has absorbed very painful experiences, has worked in service of the client for many years, and needs to be accepted, respected, and even honored. This begins the reframing process, the essence of which is helping a part of the client that once served a vital function to adapt to the "frame" of the client's current life. Therefore, instead of basing the music on the client's current state, the music is chosen to reflect the feelings and needs of the internal abuser. During the music experience, the therapist directly invites the internal abuser to surface and engage in a direct dialogue. Once the dialogue is established, the therapist guides the client's inner abuser through her or his music experience. This involves a careful mixture of normal nondirective guiding and providing the inner abuser with specific types of support and suggestion. According to Pickett and Sonnen (1993), reframing is the best and perhaps only way to engage the internal abuser in a process of change. As described earlier in reference to work with DID, the reframing technique seems to involve a significant amount of directive guiding regardless of whether a given ego is at the surface when the therapist intervenes.

Pickett and Sonnen (1993) and Pickett (1996–1997) describe the use of another type of reframing known as *phantom anchor*. This technique is used to promote healing following the re-experience of childhood trauma. Immediately following the client's re-experience and while the client is still in the music imaging, the therapist may gently hold the client's right arm or verbally state "I am here with you" and then direct the client, as his or her adult self, to be present with his/her younger, abused self in parallel (Pickett, 1996–1997). Depending on the situation and rapport between client and the imaged child, being present may include touching or holding. Once contact is established, the therapist can assist the client in communicating with the child, finding out what the child understands about what happened or what secret decision(s) he or she is making about the future in response to the trauma. The therapist can also suggest that the client comfort the child by communicating what she or he knows now but did not know then about the abuse or its aftermath. If the client is unable to do this, the therapist can offer the child comfort and make suggestions for coping and self-care. If, during the re-experiencing of trauma, the client has difficulty connecting with her or his younger self at an emotional level, the therapist directs the client to freeze the image and then employs the phantom anchor technique. Like the reframing technique, the phantom anchor technique involves directive guiding.

Gestalt Dreamwork

Clarkson (2002) discusses combining Gestalt Dreamwork with the Bonny Method. In Gestalt Dreamwork, the client first recounts an important dream slowly in an attempt to relive it in the moment; Clarkson has the client do this during the GIM prelude. Clarkson presents two types of induction that can then be used. One involves using the entire dream as an entry into further exploration similar to re-imaging. The other involves presenting objects and characters one at a time in the same succession that they appeared in the dream, allowing the client to explore each before presenting the next, as in contained spontaneous imaging. When using this latter option, the therapist is in effect providing multiple inductions throughout the music experience. During the music imaging, the client dialogues, interacts with, and/or becomes important object(s) or character(s) from her or his dream. Clarkson uses a standard GIM program and standard guiding techniques as the client explores the dream material in the music. Standard techniques are used to facilitate the postlude for Gestalt Dreamwork sessions; however, Clarkson (2002) offers additional Gestalt techniques to process the music experience of the dream material. Ones that are atypical to standard GIM practice include "empty chair" and "rehearsing" techniques. The empty chair technique involves placing an empty chair in front of the client and guiding the client to imagine that a significant person is sitting in front of him or her. The therapist then assists the client in dialoguing with the imagined person, who, in this context, would be a character from the dream. The rehearsing technique involves the therapist taking on the role of a significant person in the client's life while the client practices a new, and usually difficult, way of being in relation to this person. In the context of Gestalt Dreamwork and the Bonny Method, this would be a character from the client's dream. The use of directive guiding techniques and directive interventions (Gestalt techniques) during the postlude both represent modifications to the Bonny Method.

Music, Drawing, and Narrative

A Music, Drawing, and Narrative (MDN) session involves the client drawing to a music program and then writing about the drawing(s) while hearing the same music again (Booth, 2005–2006). An MDN session begins with a discussion of important themes, while the therapist chooses music to match the client's mood and energy. To prepare the client for the music and drawing, the therapist provides a relaxation focused on breath and support. The therapist then summarizes important themes for the client and generates a focus for the client's work. The work begins as the client moves into drawing to the music using oil pastels on 12" by 17" paper. During this phase, the therapist maintains a transcript of the drawing(s) (i.e., the sequence and relationship between colors and shapes) and the client's process as it unfolds (i.e., changes in the client's state in relation to the music). As needed, the therapist may change the music while the client draws. Once the drawing is complete, the same music used for the drawing phase is repeated to accompany the client as she or he writes the story of the drawing(s). Booth notes that the same music is used to "(1) to allow the traveler to stay immersed in the experience, (2) to time the writing, and (3) to remind the client of aspects of the experience that otherwise may be overlooked" (2005–2006, p. 57). When the client finishes writing, he or she reads the story aloud to the therapist. A dialogue ensues to further develop and ground the client's experience and to generate ideas for manifesting action outside of the session. Music programs that have been specially created for MDN sessions last from 10 to 30 minutes and contain only classical selections. To facilitate the act of drawing, the pieces have an average andante tempo, "long and organically evolving melodic lines," "varied harmonic rhythms" (Booth, 2005–2006, p. 59), and a general ABA form. Booth (2005–2006) also describes adaptations to MDN that include 50-minute sessions with shorter music programs, speaking rather than writing the story with input from the therapist, and interjecting brief GIM-like music travels. MDN seems to resemble what Bruscia (2002a) describes as projective listening, yet it includes the use of programs of classical music and seems to require the expertise of a GIM guide.

Spiritual Retreat

Holligan (1994) presents GIM sessions integrated into an individual's spiritual retreat. "A Spiritual Retreat is a period of withdrawal from normal activities to a quiet place where one can spend time in solitude, silence, and prayer. The aim is to deepen one's relationship with God and to foster spiritual growth" (p. 60). From the outset, the guide and traveler agree to this aim, and both parties agree to a prayerful approach, "to seeking the clear guidance of God's Spirit" (p. 60). A daily meeting is held to check in, perhaps discuss previous sessions, and determine whether a GIM session will be held that day. The guide may actively ask the retreatant to invite God into a discussion of important issues; however, Holligan refrains from doing this during the actual GIM sessions. Holligan recommends that at least one GIM session be conducted prior to embarking on the retreat to assess whether the client will be able to benefit from the method. Holligan's work represents a nontherapeutic use of the BMGIM and thus is a modification (Bruscia, 2002a).

Kasayka (2002) discusses a retreat format for groups designed by Clark and Kasayka. The retreats are for those interested in experiencing spirituality or connecting to God through music. Each retreat has an overarching theme such as grieving, healing, atonement, or gratitude. Sessions begin with a discussion about the difference between experiences that are psychotherapeutic and those that are spiritual or growth-oriented in nature and focus. Guidance in using the music is also provided to participants. The nature of the music imaging sessions is not specified; however, it appears that these are similar to Group GIM. The retreats include processing through expressive arts, time for personal reflection, sacred or inspirational readings, and suggestions for continued practices. This type of spiritual retreat for groups that consists of nontherapeutic goals is an example of Bonny's Group GIM (Bruscia, 2002a).

Marr (2001) presents a combination of individual and Group GIM sessions as part of a group retreat. In this format, each participant is paired with a spiritual director for individual sessions. According to Marr, spiritual direction typically involves a conversation wherein a person expresses the state of his or her spiritual journey while the director listens, accompanies, and offers guidance. Marr describes the use of individual GIM sessions in place of this discussion. In one case example, individual sessions offered by Marr were one hour in length to accommodate the retreat schedule. The preliminary discussions were focused on the retreatant's current sense of spirituality, and inductions were directed toward helping the client to connect with this in the music (e.g., "create a symbol for the presence of God within [you]," p. 402). The music imaging involved the use of one or two pieces of classical music from the GIM literature. Shortened sessions and music imaging, as well as nontherapeutic goals in individual work, are modifications of the Bonny Method (Bruscia, 2002a). A Group GIM session involved the use of one piece, Strauss's *Death and Transfiguration,* combined with a reading from the Bible (Luke 9: 28–35) regarding the Transfiguration of Christ as the starting focus. This is another example of Bonny's Group GIM.

Summary

In summary, elements of GIM have been adapted and combined with several other methods and techniques. These combined methods were not covered in the survey, but the findings related to the adaptations they contain were covered in previous chapters. Directed Imagery and Music (DIM) is like a re-imaging of a traumatic event that involves directive interventions to help the client focus on a specific life experience. DIM consists of a shortened music listening phase and no predesigned programs and may include the use of nonclassical music. Reframing during a GIM session involves the use of directive interventions and music to help clients with Dissociative Identity Disorder dialogue with their inner abuser and "reframe" or adapt to the client's current life. The phantom anchor technique during GIM involves the use of directive verbal and/or physical guiding during the music imaging to support the client in supporting his or her inner younger self following the re-experience of childhood trauma. Aspects of Gestalt Dreamwork have been used to make a client's dream the focus of a GIM session. This involves directive interventions during the prelude and postlude. Music, Drawing, and Narrative involves the client drawing and writing to short programs of classical music. During spiritual retreats, individual and Group GIM sessions have been used for the nontherapeutic purpose of helping clients to develop a deeper connection with God.

Chapter Eight

Relationships between Variations

Users of Bonny Method vs. Modifications

A key aspect of the GIM survey (Muller, 2010) was to compare the use of the BMGIM with the use of modified practices to identify any relationships that might exist. Whereas there has been disagreement regarding the boundaries of GIM practice within the GIM community and nonspecific definition of them by the AMI (Chapters Two and Nine), the survey results suggested that in practice, GIM fellows find some intrinsic value in the very boundaries established by Bruscia (2002a). Specifically, respondents who used Bonny Method practices tended not to use modified practices, and respondents who used modified practices tended not to use Bonny Method practices. Only two practices, one from each category, were positively related to each other across this boundary between practices. Specifically, respondents who use verbal dialogue during the music imaging, a Bonny Method practice, also tended to use extemporaneous programming, a modified practice. That these two are positively related seems intuitive and does not seem to sully the boundary distinctions. Therefore, what does it mean that the boundaries articulated by Bruscia (2002a) are reflected in the practices of GIM fellows? What is their clinical significance? Were these boundaries instilled into GIM fellows during their training? If this is so, it seems that some training programs favor Bonny Method practices, whereas others favor modified practices. Alternatively, to what extent were these boundaries instilled by the literature? How many GIM fellows have read and concur with Bruscia's (2002a) definitions? How might this research finding inform research, training, and practice?

Nondirective vs. Directive Interventions

The BMGIM is thought to be made up of nondirective interventions. Further comparison of practices from the survey indicated a strong positive relationship between four BMGIM practices and modified practices of the directive type. The Bonny practices in question are: (1) the use of mandalas during the prelude and postlude, (2) the use of a starting image, (3) the use of music-centered interventions, and (4) the use of physical interventions when requested by the client. This raises the question: To what extent can these practices be considered directive or nondirective? In practice, each of these four interventions has different permutations that can be placed on a continuum from nondirective to directive. Each of these relationships as indicated by the data will be summarized, followed by a discussion of each continuum.

The survey results indicated that GIM fellows who tended to use mandalas also tended to use directive interventions. Asking a client to draw a mandala during the prelude or postlude could be considered directive simply because the therapist is proposing it. However, if mandalas are introduced to the client as a regular part of the session structure, this seems unreasonable. More important is how the therapist proposes mandala use during the session. Moving along a continuum from nondirective to directive, does the therapist suggest (e.g., "Would you like to draw a mandala?"), recommend (e.g., "I think that drawing a mandala would help you to focus in preparation for the music"), or direct (e.g., "You have traveled very deeply, and I want you to draw a mandala to help you synthesize your experience").

The survey results also indicated that GIM fellows who tended to use music-centered interventions also tended to use directive guiding techniques during the music imaging and tended to use directive interventions during the prelude and postlude. As summarized in Chapter Five, Summer (2009) has studied and written extensively about music-centered interventions. She has developed an approach to GIM that involves the exclusive use of music-centered interventions that she refers to as "music-centered GIM guiding." Summer concluded that, "music-centered GIM guiding is directive, focusing essentially on the client's experience of the music" (2009, p. 115). The question at hand is: Is a single music-centered intervention directive or nondirective? It seems that music-centered interventions could be considered on at least three continua from nondirective to directive. The first continuum relates to the client's awareness of the music when the therapist intervenes. On the nondirective end of this continuum, the client is already aware of the music, perhaps reporting something about his or her music experience, and on the directive end the client is mostly unaware of the music until the guide intervenes. The second continuum relates to how the music-centered intervention is worded by the guide. On the nondirective end of this continuum, the guide suggests that the client focus on the music (e.g., "What do you notice about the music?"), and on the directive end the guide directs the client to the music (e.g., "Focus on the music now"). A third continuum relates to the degree of specificity used by the guide in reference to the music. On the nondirective end, the guide refers to the music in general as in the previous examples, and on the directive end, the guide refers to something specific (e.g., "What do you notice about the violin?"; "Do the voices have anything to communicate to you?"; "Allow the cello to resonate inside you").

The survey results indicated that GIM fellows who tended to provide a starting image also tended to introduce an image during the music. In terms of being directive, introducing an image as the music begins seems different from introducing an image after the client has been traveling within images that emerged from her or his experience of the music. Whereas both could be presented as suggestions, the latter could be perceived by the client as an intrusion. Moreover, as Bruscia (2002a) states, this type of directive intervention is typically borrowed from other orientations and is used to achieve therapeutic outcomes that emanate from outside of the client's spontaneous imaging.

Further, the survey results indicated that GIM fellows who tended to provide physical interventions when the client requests them also tended to provide physical interventions when they perceive that the client needs them. This may indicate that GIM fellows consider both types of physical interventions to be directive. As explained in Chapter Two, Bonny (2002g) discussed the use of physical interventions when the need is clearly indicated by the client. Bruscia (2002a) indicated that directive types of physical intervention that are construed by the therapist in adherence to a theoretical orientation are not related to the Bonny Method. That said, the use of a physical intervention could be construed as directive regardless of whether it emanates from the client's or the therapist's world. When the therapist uses a physical intervention, he or she has entered the client's world in a very direct way. In the altered state that occurs during music and imaging experiences, what the therapist intends to communicate and what the client perceives can easily be misconstrued, in part because the client may perceive what the therapist is feeling, and this may be amplified by physical touch (Cohen, 2002). The use of physical interventions requires the therapist to closely and carefully monitor the client–therapist relationship. Therefore, one way to understand a physical intervention as directive or nondirective is in terms of the therapist's level of clarity. In other words, the more fully the therapist makes her- or himself available to the client in the moment, the less directive the physical intervention will be. Nevertheless, even when the therapist is being fully present to the client, there are unconscious dynamics at work (Bruscia, 1998).

Discussion of directive to nondirective continua in relation to individual practices begins to illuminate the vast range of options that exist within the Bonny Method. Imagine how informative it would be to apply this and other constructs to each of the practices that make up the method.

Chapter Nine

Implications for Practice, Training, and Supervision

Levels of Practice

Variations in GIM raise the topic of levels of practice. In the literature, levels of practice are defined in terms of client functioning, practices, and music. As stated earlier, the BMGIM was originally designed for well adults, and within this context, levels of practice were already implied. In addition, the literature on the BMGIM reveals that its applications have expanded over time. As presented in Chapters Three through Seven, adapted GIM has been used to help clients with a variety of clinical concerns. Several authors indicate that adaptations are needed to accommodate fragile ego, physical frailty, limited attention span, or impaired cognition, yet the Bonny Method has been used to help clients with some of these same needs (Meadows, 2002). This raises questions: (1) Are both the BMGIM and modified GIM being used to help clients who are at the same level of functioning? (2) What criteria are fellows using to determine the need for adapted GIM over the BMGIM? (3) How are levels of practice in GIM distinguished?

Abbott (2010, 2013), Bruscia (2002d), Paik-Maier (2010, 2013) and Summer (2002, 2010) refer to three levels of practice: (1) supportive, (2) intensive or re-educative, and (3) primary or reconstructive. These levels are defined in terms of client functioning, practices, and music. Whereas descriptions of client functioning at each level are congruent among authors, the practices and music used at each level are not. Bruscia (2002d) refers to the use of GIM at all three levels. In contrast, Summer (2010) emphasizes the use of music and imagery for the first two levels and suggests that the BMGIM is best suited for clients who are ready to work at the reconstructive level. In addition, Summer (2009, 2010) suggests that individual pieces of music have either a supportive, re-educative, or reconstructive function. She states that GIM programs consist of pieces from all three of these levels (Summer, 2009). In contrast, Brucia (2002c) describes whole GIM programs in terms of "stages of traveler readiness": Beginning, Preliminary Working, Working, Advanced Working, Transpersonal. In summary, client functioning, practices, music, and music programs can be described in terms of levels of practice.

Supportive

At the supportive, level there is a need to achieve or restore internal equilibrium or congruence (Abbott, 2010; Bruscia, 2002d). At this level, the client is not ready to deal with internal or external stressors or conflicts and instead needs to focus on accessing or creating positive inner resources that will help him/her to develop ego strength (sense of self) (Abbott, 2010; Bruscia, 2002d; Summer, 2002, 2010). Moreover, the client may be able to engage only in short-term treatment and may need to work in a limited way (Bruscia, 2002d).

Supportive-level experiences are meant to be healing, but catharsis is not necessary (Bruscia, 2002d). Sessions at the supportive level are deliberately positive, "the music is easy, safe, and structure-building rather than challenging or uncovering" (Bruscia, 2002d). Programs classified by Bruscia (2002c) as "Beginning Programs" can foster supportive-level work. In addition, the therapist's approach to the prelude discussion, induction, starting image, guiding, and postlude of the BMGIM can help the client to maintain a supportive level of work. If in helping a session to be supportive for the client the therapist shortens the session or music length, uses directive interventions, or employs other than a humanistic or existential orientation, the session would be considered modified GIM.

Outside the realm of GIM, Abbott (2010), Paik-Maier (2010), and Summer (2009, 2010) describe the use of supportive music and imagery. In supportive music and imagery a single piece of music with a "simple structure and little tension" (Summer, 2010, p. 487) is played repeatedly while the client is directed to sit upright and to use pastels to explore a single image that reflects a positive experience or feeling. This highlights the dividing line between GIM and music and imagery. In supportive music and imagery, the client is in an ordinary state of consciousness. In GIM, the client freely and spontaneously explores his/her inner world in an expanded state of consciousness. Supportive music and imagery involves the use of music-centered programming combined with directive interventions to keep the client focused on a single positive image. Alone or in combination, these two practices could fall within the boundary of modified GIM. It is the added direction to sit upright and draw in an ordinary state of consciousness that moves the practice outside of the GIM boundary.

Intensive (Re-educative)

At the intensive level, the client is ready to work on making changes within his/her inner world and to engage any incongruence, tensions, or difficult emotions that arise in the process (Abbott, 2010). At this level, the client can directly engage internal issues or problems that impact multiple areas of life and develop insights that s/he can apply outside of sessions (Abbott, 2010; Bruscia, 2002d; Summer, 2002, 2010). Here the client is able to work for a more sustained period (Bruscia, 2002d).

Intensive-level experiences are designed "to help the client to uncover, work through, and gain insight" (Bruscia, 2002d). The client–therapist relationship is important here, as is the verbal processing needed to help clients to integrate their experiences (Abbott, 2010; Bruscia, 2002d; Summer, 2010). Bruscia (2002d) suggests that intensive-level work include eight or more individual GIM sessions, which may be accompanied by couple or Group GIM sessions with therapeutic goals for the client. Music programs classified by Bruscia (2002c) as "Preliminary Working Programs" can foster intensive-level work. As with supportive-level work, the phases of the BMGIM session can be made to suit the client's needs at the intensive level. If this involves shortening the session or music length, using directive interventions, or other than a humanistic or existential orientation, the work would be considered modified GIM.

Beyond the GIM boundary, Abbott (2010) and Summer (2009, 2010) describe the use of re-educative music and imagery. Summer (2010) explains that this level of music and imagery includes "inductions with repetitive music that matches the [client's] symptom with harmonic tension, but contains little structural development" (p. 486). As with music and imagery at the supportive level, the client is directed to focus on a single image and draw to the music while sitting upright (Abbott, 2010). Here again, the dividing line between GIM and music and imagery is illuminated. During both the supportive and re-educative levels of music and imagery, the client is in an ordinary state of consciousness.

Primary (Reconstructive)

At the primary level, the client is healthy enough to address problems at their core and to experience more profound shifts in consciousness (Bruscia, 2002d; Summer, 2009, 2010). At this level, the need for insight and generalization is diminished as the client can in the moment delve into the "unconscious roots of existing emotional tensions and … into existential and spiritual questions" (Summer, 2009, p. 84), release old ways, and integrate new ways of being.

Primary-level experiences are essentially transformative. Bruscia (2002d) imparts, "The goal is to remove limits of imagination which in turn expands and deepens experience, which in turn changes the relationship between the person and his world" (p. 6). Bruscia (2002d) and Summer (2009, 2010) refer to the use of the BMGIM at this level, and some forms of modified GIM may also be indicated. Music programs classified by Bruscia (2002c) as "Working," "Advanced Working," and "Transpersonal" can foster work at the primary level. A reconstructive form of music and imagery has not been identified in the literature.

Modifications: Skill Levels

Variations in GIM practice raise the question, Are there levels of skill with regard to specific Bonny Method or modified practices? Bruscia (2002c) refers to three levels of music programming in GIM: basic, intermediate, and advanced. At the basic level, the guide uses a predesigned program without making changes, moves from one predesigned program to another as needed, or adds pieces to the end of a program from a list of recommended "tags." At the intermediate level, the guide spontaneously chooses from a group of pieces that have been pregrouped together or spontaneously chooses portions of different predesigned programs and sequences them together. At the advanced level, in addition to having the expertise to program extemporaneously without constraint, the guide is a creator of GIM programs. A fellow qualified at this level designs programs or groupings of pieces for their own use or for the use of others in GIM. Summer's (2009) music-centered programming seems to correspond to the intermediate and/or advanced levels here.

Summer (2009) refers to both her music-centered programming and music-centered guiding as advanced practices. Can skill levels be further articulated for music-centered or other types of guiding? Are there skill levels for other Bonny Method or modified practices that are yet to be articulated?

Variations in Training and Supervision

Traditionally, training in the BMGIM has been divided into three levels (Lewis, 2002). At the first two levels, trainees become familiar with the method through didactic learning, observing demo sessions, experiencing the BMGIM as a client, and practicing the method under close supervision. Trainees who reach the third level practice the method more extensively and learn about "advanced concepts." This learning may include modified forms of GIM (AMI, 2010), which seem to vary with the experience and interests of the trainer (e.g., extemporaneous programming, psychodynamic orientation, physical interventions initiated by the therapist). It is unclear whether training in modified forms of GIM includes personal experiences as a client or supervised practice in their use (AMI, 2010).

In recent years, new training models that incorporate training in music and imagery have emerged in the United States (Abbott, 2010, 2013; Montgomery, 2010; Paik-Maier, 2010, 2013) and in Europe (Abbott, 2010). In some cases, supportive and re-educative music and imagery are used as a precursor to training in the Bonny Method (Abbott, 2010, 2013; Paik-Maier, 2013); in other cases, music and imagery training is separate from GIM training (Therapeutic Arts Institute, 2013). As in GIM training, in addition to learning how to practice music and imagery, trainees are required to have personal music and imagery sessions and to be supervised in its use. In each of these cases, it is GIM fellows who are teaching others how to use music and imagery.

These variations raise questions. Should some degree of mastery of the BMGIM precede training and practice of modified GIM? Can the reverse be true? What about music and imagery? In learning the BMGIM, is being a client in modified GIM as informative as being a client in the BMGIM or vice versa? What about music and imagery? Can modified GIM be safely and effectively used without prior supervised practice and personal experience?

Use of Terms

It is important that the BMGIM, modified GIM, and music and imagery be clearly distinguished from one another (Abbott, 2013; Bruscia, 2002a; Summer, 2009). Practices that fall into these three categories require different levels of training, are intended for different purposes, and have different therapeutic potentials. Unclear distinction between these practices can compromise professionals', students', and clients' ability to make ethical and healthy decisions about them. Over the past decade, some forms of music and imagery have been referred to as modifications of the Bonny Method. Whereas some forms of music and imagery may have been inspired or informed by the BMGIM, they clearly fall outside the boundaries of GIM practice (Bruscia, 2002a; Summer, 2009). Practices that fall outside the boundary of the BMGIM but remain within the boundary of GIM have most often been referred to as modifications or adaptations of the Bonny Method, or simply modified GIM. Referring to music and imagery practices as a modification of the Bonny Method can mislead readers to think that music and imagery practices belong to GIM.

The potential for such confusion is compounded by the advent of trainings that include instruction in both GIM and music and imagery. According to the American Music Therapy Association (2008) Professional Competencies and the Certification Board for Music Therapists (2008) Scope of Practice, music therapists are educated and trained in music and imagery and use it in practice. Should forms of music and imagery that are taught by GIM fellows and can lead to training in the BMGIM be distinguished from other forms of music and imagery that are taught by music therapists who are not trained in the BMGIM? If there are forms of music and imagery that the GIM community feels require specific training that exceeds the standards set for music therapists by the AMTA, they should be specified to ensure safe and ethical practice. Add to this the practice of Guided Music Imaging (GMI), a type of "imaginal listening" briefly mentioned by Bruscia (1998) that is detailed in the music therapy literature by Grocke and Wigram (2007). These authors use the term GMI to refer to adaptations of the BMGIM that involve a shortened, 1½-hour session and 10 to 20 minutes of music. Is this the beginning of a new set of acronyms to label different types of modifications? Grocke and Wigram (2007) recommend a minimum of Level I or Level II GIM training to practice GMI. It seems clear that GMI is modified GIM, but is it also being presented as a form of music and imagery that can be practiced by music therapists who have not received training under the AMI?

Regardless, if it is important to differentiate GIM from music and imagery (Abbott, 2013; Bruscia, 2002a; Summer, 2009), then music and imagery cannot at the same time be both a modification of the BMGIM or modified GIM and not GIM. In addition, it seems important that trainees in programs where music and imagery is used as a precursor to training in the BMGIM *not* be referred to as "GIM trainees" until they reach the third level. The same holds for reference to the training programs themselves, as trainees may well leave after completing one or two levels and not be trained in GIM at all.

To date there have been only two publications where the terms BMGIM, modified GIM, and music and imagery are clearly differentiated (Bruscia, 2002a; Muller, 2010). "Core Elements" of the BMGIM are defined in the AMI Standards (2010), as are "Core Elements" of training in the BMGIM, but they do not include criteria for distinguishing between the BMGIM, modified GIM, and music and imagery. In their present form, these core elements can easily be construed as referring to each of these practices, including the supportive and re-educative music and imagery described earlier. Whereas the AMI standards (2010) imply that training should primarily be focused on the BMGIM, without a clear definition of what the BMGIM is and what it is not, how can trainers or students know the difference?

Chapter Ten

Summary

This chapter includes summary and discussion of Chapters Three through Six and the boundaries of practice with implications, recommendations, and closing thoughts.

Length of Session and Music

As of 2009, the standard session lasting 1½ to 2 hours with 30 minutes or more of music was still in use by a majority of practitioners. Music lengths of 21 to 30 minutes are also widely used. Shortened session lengths and music imaging were being used in individual sessions with psychiatric, physically ill, and child clients, but much less so than the Bonny Method standard. Sessions and music were shortened to accommodate individual client needs (fragile ego, physical frailty, limited attention span). Session length has also been shortened to accommodate therapist or facility scheduling. GIM fellows outside the United States used a 1½- to 2-hour session more often than those in the United States. The use of certain Bonny Method and modified session and music lengths seemed to vary in relation to practitioners' work with certain client age groups and client concerns in ways that were consistent with the literature. Further research is needed to confirm these and other relationships that may exist between length of session, population, conditions, goal, and characteristics of practitioners.

Selection and Use of Music

As of 2009, a majority of practitioners were still using the standard predesigned music programs containing classical music. Practitioners were also practicing extemporaneous programming and using nonclassical music, but much less so than the Bonny Method standard. For psychologically or physically fragile clients, nonclassical music was used to limit the expansion and exploration of consciousness; more often, however, consonant and structured classical music were used to have this same effect. Extemporaneous programming was used to respond to the client's in-the-moment needs. A new "music-centered" approach to programming has been created to limit the generation of imagery while deepening the client's experience of the music. The use of certain Bonny Method and modified types of music and approaches to programming seemed to vary in relation to work with certain client age groups and client concerns in ways that are consistent with the literature. Further research is needed to confirm relationships that may exist between types of programming and between types of music and length of session, population, conditions, goal, and characteristics of practitioners.

Verbal Dialogue and Guiding

As of 2009, a nondirective approach to verbal dialogue and music imaging was still being used by a majority of practitioners, as were the standard dialogue during the music imaging, music-centered interventions, and physical interventions when requested by the client. Directive interventions, including introducing an image during the music experience, physical interventions when the need is perceived by the therapist, having the client sit in an upright position during the music imaging, and having the client image with eyes open, were also reported but much less so than the Bonny Method standard. Directive interventions were used to limit the expansion and exploration of consciousness, to provide clients with immediate reinforcement, and to guide clients toward positive experiences. A new "music-centered" approach to guiding has been created to focus the client's awareness on the music and away from the imagery. GIM fellows within the United States used physical interventions when they perceived the client needed them more often than those outside the United States. The use of certain Bonny Method and modified verbal and physical interventions seemed to vary in relation to work with certain client age groups and client concerns. Some of these had support in the literature, while some did not. Further research is needed to confirm relationships that may exist between types of verbal dialogue and guiding and population, conditions, goal, and characteristics of practitioners.

Theoretical Orientation

As of 2009, humanistic/existential was the preferred theoretical orientation of practitioners, followed by psychodynamic, transpersonal/spiritual, and Jungian. Very few practitioners preferred bioenergetic, somatic, and/or chakra or cognitive/behavioral and no practitioners preferred Gestalt as their primary orientation; however, each of these orientations was used during the prelude, music imaging, and postlude. In contrast to other categories, here the gap between the use of Bonny Method and modified orientations, specifically psychodynamic and Jungian, is not nearly as wide. Adopting a particular theoretical orientation is significant, as it influences every decision that a therapist makes on behalf of the client, and this may include modified interventions. The use of certain Bonny Method and modified theoretical orientations seemed to vary in relation to work with certain client age groups and client concerns. There was no direct support for this in the literature. Further research is needed to confirm relationships that may exist between theoretical orientations and population, conditions, goal, and characteristics of practitioners.

Bonny Method Practices and Modifications

The results of the survey indicated that each of the following four defining Bonny Method practices (Bruscia, 2002a) were in frequent use by a majority (more than 75%) of GIM fellows: (1) 1½- to 2-hour session, (2) 30 minutes or more of music for a 1½- to 2-hour session, (3) verbal dialogue during the music imaging, and (4) predesigned programs. The use of theoretical orientations (humanistic/existential or transpersonal/spiritual) attributed to the BMGIM (Bruscia, 2002) was less prevalent, with only 50% of respondents reporting that they use them at least "often." Viewing these Bonny Method practices and theoretical orientations as a group, nearly half of the respondents reported using all four of the practices at least "often," whereas just over one quarter of respondents reported also using a theoretical orientation consistent with the Bonny Method. Based on the current data, it seems that the use of the structural elements of the Bonny Method is more important to GIM fellows than the use of a humanistic/existential or transpersonal/spiritual orientation. There is no apparent explanation for this. Applying Bruscia's (2002a) distinctions here, it seems that only 25% of GIM fellows are practicing the Bonny Method of Guided Imagery and Music in full "often" or "always." According the AMI (2010) standards, GIM training is focused on learning to use the BMGIM; however, the specific practices that constitute the BMGIM are not specified, and no reference is made to Bruscia's (2002a) or any definition of what constitutes the Bonny Method. To what extent are GIM trainers teaching the use of the four practices listed above? To what extent are humanistic/existential or transpersonal/spiritual orientations taught?

On the Relationships between Variations

A very interesting finding of the survey is that there appear to be two distinct groups of GIM practitioners: those who tended to use the Bonny Method as originally conceived for most of their clientele and those who tended to modify the method (see Chapter Eight). Further, those who used the original method tended not to modify it, and those who modified it tended not to use the original method. It is vital that this relationship be further investigated and understood as it relates to training and practice.

Another interesting finding is that there seems to be a correlation between level of directiveness and the use of certain practices. Specifically, practitioners who used directive interventions tended to use mandalas, starting images, music-centered interventions, and physical interventions when requested by the client. An important revelation here is that there are likely vast differences among practitioners regarding degrees of directiveness. This was not taken into account in the survey and could be the source of an entirely new study of variations in GIM.

Implications

Variations in GIM practice raise several important issues. The first is that there seem to be differences of opinion among the GIM community as to what constitutes a variation or modification to the original method. In contrast, the survey data indicated that GIM fellows recognize, at least tacitly, the same boundaries articulated by Bruscia (2002a). This contradiction needs to be investigated. In addition, there is no denying that the BMGIM was developed through extensive research (Summer, 2002d). Modifications to the BMGIM need to be researched separately.

The second issue is that according to the AMI Standards (2010), GIM training is primarily focused on the BMGIM, and yet the survey revealed that only half of practitioners are practicing it in full. To what extent are GIM trainers teaching the structural elements of the BMGIM alone or in combination? To what extent are they teaching the use of humanistic/existential or transpersonal/spiritual orientations? What about modifications? Note that transference and countertransference dynamics increase as interventions become more directive (Bruscia, 1998c; Grocke, 1995). Are trainers that emphasize modifications also instructing trainees to work psychodynamically? Bruscia (2002c) and Summer (2009) define some modified practices (e.g., spontaneous programming; music-centered guiding) as advanced. According to the AMI (2010), advanced practices are covered during Level III GIM training. Is this enough? Should further requirements for training in or the use of these or other modifications be specified? All of these boundaries are important; without them, it is unclear who is trained to do what, what practices are potentially harmful when used by the untrained, and what practices can be used safely to benefit patients.

The third issue is that there seem to be differences of opinion as to why specific variations are needed. Some practitioners relate the need for variations to specific client needs (e.g., fragile ego, impaired cognition). Others relate variations to the level of practice most appropriate for the client (e.g., supportive, re-educative, reconstructive), while others vary to accommodate personal styles (e.g., theoretical orientation) or situations (e.g., scheduling). These different rationales raise fundamental questions about the nature of GIM training and call for further investigation.

Closing Thoughts

After being immersed in this material for several years, I wonder why the GIM community seems unready to accept that boundaries exist between the various practices and unready to accept the need to clearly define and differentiate them. What is with all the resistance and fracturing? The advent of modifications need *not* signal the end of the Bonny Method, and rediscovering the Bonny Method and articulating its ever subtle aspects need *not* compromise the discovery of modifications. If the survey of GIM fellows revealed anything, it revealed that the two can serve a vital role in informing each other, but only if we remain open and thoughtful.

The truth is that all of the variations were born out of Helen Bonny's discovery and the method that she created. What represents true mastery of the BMGIM? Has anyone achieved this? I think not. The beauty of a method, or more accurately a *model* (Bruscia, 1998a), like Helen's is that it morphs to suit the style of each practitioner, and in the hands of the competent practitioner, it morphs to meet the needs of each individual client. There are as many ways to use it as there are practitioners to learn it. No one person can fully understand or master the Bonny Method, nor could Bonny! Another one of the inherent values of the BMGIM is that it contains procedures to help the therapist to weed out aspects of her or his own influence that may impede the client's progress (e.g., dialoguing with the client, being nondirective, hearing the music as the client hears it, maintaining a written transcript). To what extent is this inherent value retained in the modifications? Models like the BMGIM are rare and unique, and this elevates the need to clearly define and understand them in their original state. I believe that there is much more to learn about the BMGIM and that continued investigation of it is the primary path to understanding modifications to it.

Summary

There are myriad paths to the divine and myriad degrees to which a human being can open to it through the music and through relationship. Nearly 12 years into being a GIM fellow, I marvel at how accommodating the BMGIM is and how different it is each time for each person. The LSD was pushy; the BMGIM is accepting yet challenging, gentle yet powerful, subtle yet profound, and, when I am truly there for the client and not in the way, healing, in that vitally personal way.

References

Abbott, E. (2010). The Bonny Method: Training innovations at Anna Maria College. *Voices: A World Forum for Music Therapy, 10*(3). Retrieved November 16, 2013, from https://normt.uib.no/index.php/voices/article/view/501/424

Abbott, E. (2013). Music and imagery self-experience in the clinical supervision of trainees in Guided Imagery and Music. In K. E. Bruscia (Ed.), *Self experiences in music therapy education, training, and supervision* (pp. 866–899). University Park, IL: Barcelona Publishers.

Abrams, B. (2002). Definitions of transpersonal BMGIM experience. *Nordic Journal of Music Therapy, 11*(2), 103–126.

Abrams, B. (Ed.). (2004, Winter/Spring). Results of editor's survey. *Bonny Method Resources, 17*, 1–2.

American Music Therapy Association. (2008). *AMTA professional competencies.* Silver Spring, MD: Author.

Association for Music and Imagery. (2010). *Manual of standards and procedures for endorsement of the Bonny Method of GIM trainers and training programs* (Revised September, 2010). Blaine, WA: Author.

Association for Music and Imagery. (2009). *2009 fellows registry.* Blaine, WA: Author.

Association for Music and Imagery. (2010). The Bonny Method: General information. Retrieved May 10, 2010, from: http://www.ami-bonnymethod.org /general_information.asp. Blaine, WA: Author.

Blake, R. L. (1994). Vietnam veterans with post-traumatic stress disorder: Findings from a music and imagery project. *Journal of the Association for Music and Imagery, 3*, 5–17.

Blake, R. L., & Bishop, S. R. (1994). The Bonny Method of Guided Imagery and Music (GIM) in the treatment of post-traumatic stress disorder (PTSD) with adults in the psychiatric setting. *Music Therapy Perspectives, 12*(2), 125–129.

Bonny, H. L. (2002a). Autobiographical essay. In L. Summer (Ed.), *Music and consciousness: The evolution of Guided Imagery and Music* (pp. 1–18). University Park, IL: Barcelona Publishers.

Bonny, H. L. (2002b). Discovery of the method. In L. Summer (Ed.), *Music and consciousness: The evolution of Guided Imagery and Music* (pp. 43–52). University Park, IL: Barcelona Publishers.

Bonny, H. L. (2002c). The early development of GIM. In L. Summer (Ed.), *Music and consciousness: The evolution of Guided Imagery and Music* (pp. 53–68). University Park, IL: Barcelona Publishers.

Bonny, H. L. (2002d). The role of taped music programs in the Guided Imagery and Music (GIM) process. In L. Summer (Ed.), *Music and consciousness: The evolution of Guided Imagery and Music* (pp. 299–324). University Park, IL: Barcelona Publishers.

Bonny, H. L. (2002e). Twenty-one years later: A GIM update. In L. Summer (Ed.), *Music and consciousness: The evolution of Guided Imagery and Music* (pp. 141–154). University Park, IL: Barcelona Publishers.

Bonny, H. L. (2002f). Music and spirituality. In L. Summer (Ed.), *Music and consciousness: The evolution of Guided Imagery and Music* (pp. 175–184). University Park, IL: Barcelona Publishers.

Bonny, H. L. (2002g). Facilitating Guided Imagery and Music (GIM) sessions. In L. Summer (Ed.), *Music and consciousness: The evolution of Guided Imagery and Music* (pp. 269–298). University Park, IL: Barcelona Publishers.

Bonny, H. L. (2002h). Founding the Institute for Consciousness and Music (ICM). In L. Summer (Ed.), *Music and consciousness: The evolution of Guided Imagery and Music* (pp. 69–76). University Park, IL: Barcelona Publishers.

Bonny, H. L., & Goldberg, F. S. (2002). New directions in the Bonny Method of Guided Imagery and Music. In L. Summer (Ed.), *Music and consciousness: The evolution of Guided Imagery and Music* (pp. 263–268). University Park, IL: Barcelona Publishers.

References

Bonny, H. L., & Keiser Mardis, L. (1994). *Music resources for GIM facilitators: Core programs and discography of core programs.* Olney, MD: Archedigm Publications.

Booth, J. M. (1998–1999). The paradise program: A new music program for Guided Imagery and Music. *Journal of the Association for Music and Imagery, 6,* 15–35.

Booth, J. M. (2005–2006). Music, drawing, and narrative: An adaptation of the Bonny Method of Guided Imagery and Music. *Journal of the Association for Music and Imagery, 10,* 55–73.

Brooks, D. M. (2000). Anima manifestations of men using Guided Imagery and Music: A case study. *Journal of the Association for Music and Imagery, 7,* 77–87.

Bruscia, K. E. (1991). Embracing life with AIDS: Psychotherapy through Guided Imagery and Music (GIM). In K. E. Bruscia (Ed.), *Case studies in music therapy.* University Park, IL: Barcelona Publishers.

Bruscia, K. E. (1995). Manifestations of transference in Guided Imagery and Music. *Journal of the Association for Music and Imagery, 4,* 17–36.

Bruscia, K. E. (1998a). *Defining music therapy* (2nd ed.). University Park, IL: Barcelona Publishers.

Bruscia, K. E. (1998b). An introduction to music psychotherapy. In K. E. Bruscia (Ed.), *The dynamics of music psychotherapy* (pp. 1–16). University Park, IL: Barcelona Publishers.

Bruscia, K. E. (1998c). Modes of consciousness in guided imagery and music: A therapist's experience of the guiding process. In K. E. Bruscia (Ed.), *The dynamics of music psychotherapy* (pp. 491–526). University Park, IL: Barcelona Publishers.

Bruscia, K. E. (2000). The nature of meaning in music therapy. *Nordic Journal of Music Therapy, 9*(2), 84–96.

Bruscia, K. E. (2002a). The boundaries of Guided Imagery and Music (GIM) and the Bonny Method. In K. E. Bruscia & D. E. Grocke (Eds.), *Guided Imagery and Music: The Bonny Method and beyond* (pp. 37–61). University Park, IL: Barcelona Publishers.

Bruscia, K. E. (2002b). A psychodynamic orientation to the bonny method. In K. E. Bruscia & D. E. Grocke (Eds.), *Guided Imagery and Music: The Bonny Method and beyond* (pp. 225–244). University Park, IL: Barcelona Publishers.

Bruscia, K. E. (2002c). Developments in programming for the Bonny Method. In K. E. Bruscia & D. E. Grocke (Eds.), *Guided Imagery and Music: The Bonny Method and beyond* (pp. 307–315). University Park, IL: Barcelona Publishers.

Bruscia, K. E. (2002d). *A Manual for Introductory (Level One) Training in Guided Imagery and Music.* Unpublished manuscript.

Bruscia, K. E. (2003). *Discography of GIM programs.* Unpublished manuscript.

Bruscia, K. E., & Grocke, D. E. (2002). Appendices C–L: Music Programs for Guided Imagery and Music (GIM). In K. E. Bruscia & D. E. Grocke (Eds.), *Guided Imagery and Music: The Bonny Method and beyond* (pp. 563–591). University Park, IL: Barcelona Publishers.

Burns, D. S. (2002). Guided Imagery and Music (GIM) in the treatment of individuals with chronic illnesses. In K. E. Bruscia & D. E. Grocke (Eds.), *Guided Imagery and Music: The Bonny Method and beyond* (pp. 171–186). University Park, IL: Barcelona Publishers.

Certification Board for Music Therapists. (2010). *Certification Board for Music Therapists Scope of Practice, effective October 2010.* Downingtown, PA: Author.

Clark, M. F. (1991). Emergence of the adult self in Guided Imagery and Music (GIM) therapy. In K. E. Bruscia (Ed.), *Case studies in music therapy* (pp. 321–332). University Park, IL: Barcelona Publishers.

Clark, M. F. (2002). Evolution of the Bonny Method of Guided Imagery and Music (GIM). In K. E. Bruscia & D. E. Grocke (Eds.), *Guided Imagery and Music: The Bonny Method and beyond* (pp. 5–27). University Park, IL: Barcelona Publishers.

Clarkson, G. (1995). Adapting a Guided Imagery and Music series for a nonverbal man with autism. *Journal of the Association for Music and Imagery, 4,* 121–138.

Clarkson, G. (2002). Combining Gestalt dreamwork and the Bonny Method. In K. E. Bruscia & D. E. Grocke (Eds.), *Guided Imagery and Music: The Bonny Method and beyond* (pp. 245–256). University Park, IL: Barcelona Publishers.

Clarkson, G., & Geller, J. D. (1996). The Bonny Method from a psychoanalytic perspective: Insights from working with a psychoanalytic psychotherapist in a Guided Imagery and Music series. *The Arts in Psychotherapy, 23*(4), 311–319.

Cohen, N. (2002). Ethical considerations in Guided Imagery and Music. In K. E. Bruscia & D. E. Grocke (Eds.), *Guided Imagery and Music: The Bonny Method and beyond* (pp. 483–495). University Park, IL: Barcelona Publishers.

Ducette, J. (2010). *Factor analysis.* Unpublished manuscript, Department of Educational Psychology, Temple University, Philadelphia, PA.

Goldberg, F. S. (1994). The Bonny Method of Guided Imagery and Music as individual and group treatment in a short-term acute psychiatric hospital. *Journal of the Association for Music and Imagery, 3,* 18–34.

Goldberg, F. S., Hoss, T. M., & Chesna, T. (1988). Music and imagery as psychotherapy with a brain-damaged patient: A case study. *Music Therapy Perspectives, 5,* 41–45.

Grinder, J., & Bandler, R. (1981). *Tranceformations.* Moab, UT: Real People Press.

Grocke, D. E. (2002a). The evolution of Bonny's music programs. In K. E. Bruscia & D. E. Grocke (Eds.), *Guided Imagery and Music: The Bonny Method and beyond* (pp. 85–98). University Park, IL: Barcelona Publishers.

Grocke, D. E. (2002b). The Bonny music programs. In K. E. Bruscia & D. E. Grocke (Eds.), *Guided Imagery and Music: The Bonny Method and beyond* (pp. 99–133). University Park, IL: Barcelona Publishers.

Grocke, D. E. (2002c). International advances in Guided Imagery and Music (GIM). In K. E. Bruscia & D. E. Grocke (Eds.), *Guided Imagery and Music: The Bonny Method and beyond* (pp. 533–546). University Park, IL: Barcelona Publishers.

Grocke, D. E. (2005). The role of the therapist in the Bonny Method of Guided Imagery and Music. *Music Therapy Perspectives, 23*(1), 45–52.

Grocke, D. E., & Wigram, T. (2007). Music, visualizations and imagery. In D. E. Grocke & T. Wigram (Eds.), *Receptive methods in music therapy: Techniques and clinical applications for music therapy clinicians, educators and students* (pp. 127–156). London: Jessica Kingsley.

Hahna, N. D., & Borling, J. E. (2003–2004). The Bonny Method of Guided Imagery and Music (BMGIM) with intimate partner violence (IPV). *Journal of the Association for Music and Imagery, 9*, 41–57.

Holligan, F. (1992). Case study: Guided imagery and music. *Australian Journal of Music Therapy, 3*, 35–41.

Holligan, F. (1994). Guided Imagery and Music in spiritual retreat. *Journal of the Association for Music and Imagery, 3*, 59–68.

Isenberg-Grzeda, C. (1998). Transference structures in Guided Imagery and Music. In K. E. Bruscia (Ed.), *The dynamics of music psychotherapy* (pp. 461–480). University Park, IL: Barcelona Publishers.

Johnson, D. (1987). The role of the creative arts therapies in the diagnosis and treatment of psychological trauma. *The Arts in Psychotherapy, 14*(1), 7–13.

Kachigan, S. K. (1991). *Multivariate statistical analysis* (2nd ed.). New York, NY: Radius Press.

Kagin, R. (2010). *The relationship between music therapists' spiritual beliefs and clinical practice.* Unpublished doctoral dissertation. Temple University, Philadelphia, PA.

Kasayka, R. (2002). A spiritual orientation to the Bonny Method: To walk the mystical path on practical feet. In K. E. Bruscia & D. E. Grocke (Eds.), *Guided Imagery and Music: The Bonny Method and beyond* (pp. 257–272). University Park, IL: Barcelona Publishers.

Keiser Mardis, L. (1986). *Conscious Listening: An Annotated Guide to the ICM Taped Music Programs.* Olney, MD: Archedigm Publications.

Keiser Mardis, L. (1996). *Program 33: A new program and a new programming concept.* Olney, MD: Archedigm Publications.

Korlin, D. (2002). A neuropsychological theory of traumatic imagery in the Bonny Method of Guided Imagery and Music (BMGIM). In K. E. Bruscia & D. E. Grocke (Eds.), *Guided imagery and music: The Bonny method and beyond* (pp. 379–416). University Park, IL: Barcelona Publishers.

Korlin, D. (2007-2008). Breath grounding and modulation of the Bonny Method of Guided Imagery and Music (GIM): Theory, method, and consecutive cases. *Journal of the Association for Music and Imagery, 11,* 79-113.

Lewis, L. (2002). The development of training in the Bonny Method of Guided Imagery and Music (BMGIM) from 1975 to 2000. In K. E. Bruscia & D. E. Grocke (Eds.), *Guided imagery and music: The Bonny method and beyond* (pp. 497–517). University Park, IL: Barcelona Publishers.

Marr, J. (1998–1999). GIM at the end of life: Case studies in palliative care. *Journal of the Association for Music and Imagery, 6,* 37–54.

Marr, J. (2001). The use of the Bonny Method of Guided Imagery and Music (GIM) in spiritual growth. *The Journal of Pastoral Care, 55*(4), 397–406.

Meadows, A. (2002). Psychotherapeutic applications of the Bonny Method. In K. E. Bruscia & D. E. Grocke (Eds.), *Guided Imagery and Music: The Bonny Method and beyond* (pp. 187–204). University Park, IL: Barcelona Publishers.

Moe, T. (2002). Restitutional factors in receptive group music therapy inspired by GIM. *Nordic Journal of Music Therapy, 11*(2), 152–166.

Moe, T. (2011-2012). Group guided imagery and music therapy for inpatients with substance abuse disorder. *Journal of the Association for Music and Imagery, 13,* 78-98.

Moe, T., Roesen, A., & Raben, H. (2000). Restitutional factors in group music therapy with psychiatric patients based on a modification of Guided Imagery and Music (GIM). *Nordic Journal of Music Therapy, 9*(2), 36–50.

Moffitt, L., & Hall, A. (2003–2004). "New grown with pleasant pain" (Keats): Recovering from sexual abuse with the use of the bonny method of Guided Imagery and Music and the use of poetry. *Journal of the Association for Music and Imagery, 9,* 59–77.

Montgomery, E. (2012). The Bonny Method: Training innovations at Anna Maria College. *Voices: A World Forum for Music Therapy, 10*(3). Retrieved November 16, 2013, from: https://voices.no/index.php/voices/issue/view/71

Muller, B. J. (2010). Guided Imagery and Music: A survey of current practices. Doctoral dissertation. Temple University, Philadelphia, PA. *Dissertation Abstracts International, 71.*

Murphy, K. (2008). The effect of group Guided Imagery and Music on the psychological health of adults in substance abuse treatment. Doctoral dissertation. Temple University, Philadelphia, PA. *Dissertation Abstracts International, 69.*

Pellitteri, J. S. (1998). A self-analysis of transference in Guided Imagery and Music. In K. E. Bruscia (Ed.), The *dynamics of music psychotherapy* (pp. 481–490). University Park, IL: Barcelona Publishers.

Pickett, E. (1996–1997). Guided Imagery and Music in head trauma rehabilitation. *Journal of the Association for Music and Imagery, 5,* 51–60.

Pickett, E., & Sonnen, C. (1993). Guided Imagery and Music: A music therapy approach to multiple personality disorder. *Journal of the Association for Music and Imagery, 2,* 49–72.

Powell, L. T. (2007–2008). An adaptation of the Bonny Method of Guided Imagery and Music for public schools. *Journal of the Association for Music and Imagery, 11,* 65–78.

Ritchey Vaux, D. (1993). GIM applied to the 50-minute hour. *Journal of the Association for Music and Imagery, 2,* 29–34.

Roy, M. (1996–1997). Guided Imagery and Music group experiences with adolescent girls in a high school setting. *Journal of the Association for Music and Imagery, 5,* 61–74.

Short, A. E. (1992). Music and imagery with physically disabled elderly residents: A GIM adaptation. *Music Therapy, 11*(1), 65–98.

Short, A. E. (1996–1997). Jungian archetypes in GIM therapy: Approaching the client's fairy tale. *Journal of the Association for Music and Imagery, 5,* 37–50.

Short, A. E. (1999). At the heart of the matter: Communicating underlying messages through music and imagery in cardiac care. In R. R. Pratt & D. E. Grocke (Eds.), *Music medicine 3: Music medicine and music therapy: Expanding horizons* (pp. 313–323). St. Louis, MO: MMB Music, Inc.

Short, A. E. (2002). Guided Imagery and Music (GIM) in medical care. In K. E. Bruscia & D. E. Grocke (Eds.), *Guided Imagery and Music: The Bonny Method and beyond* (pp. 151–170). University Park, IL: Barcelona Publishers.

Short, A. E. (2007). Theme and variations on quietness: Relaxation-focused music and imagery in aged care. *Australian Journal of Music Therapy, 18,* 39–61.

Skaggs, R. (1997a). *Finishing strong: Treating chemical addictions with music and imagery.* St. Louis, MO: MMB Music.

Skaggs, R. (1997b). Music-centered creative arts in a sex offender treatment program for male juveniles. *Music Therapy Perspectives, 15*(2), 73–78.

Smith, B. (1996–1997). Uncovering and healing hidden wounds: Using GIM to resolve complicated and disenfranchised grief. *Journal of the Association for Music and Imagery, 5,* 13–36.

Summer, L. (1981). Guided Imagery and Music with the elderly. *Music Therapy, 1*(1), 39–42.

Summer, L. (1988). *Guided Imagery and Music in the institutional setting.* St. Louis, MO: MMB Music, Inc.

Summer, L. (1992). Music: The aesthetic elixir. *Journal of the Association for Music and Imagery, 1,* 43–54.

Summer, L. (1995). Melding musical and psychological processes: The therapeutic musical space. *Journal of the Association for Music and Imagery, 4,* 37–48.

Summer, L. (1998). The pure music transference in Guided Imagery and Music. In K. E. Bruscia (Ed.), *The dynamics of music psychotherapy* (pp. 431–460). University Park, IL: Barcelona Publishers.

Summer, L. (2002a). Editor's notes. In L. Summer (Ed.), *Music consciousness: The evolution of Guided Imagery and Music* (pp. 51–52). University Park, IL: Barcelona Publishers.

Summer, L. (2002b). Editor's notes. In L. Summer (Ed.), *Music consciousness: The evolution of Guided Imagery and Music* (p. 176). University Park, IL: Barcelona Publishers.

Summer, L. (2002c). Group music and imagery therapy: Emergent receptive techniques in music therapy practice. In K. E. Bruscia & D. E. Grocke (Eds.), *Guided Imagery and Music: The Bonny Method and beyond* (pp. 297–306). University Park, IL: Barcelona Publishers.

Summer, L. (2009). *Client perspectives on the music in Guided Imagery and Music.* Doctoral dissertation. Retrieved from http://www.mt-phd.aau.dk/resources/ phd_dissertations

Summer, L. (2010). Music therapy and depression: Uncovering resources in music and imagery. In A. Meadows (Ed.), *Developments in music therapy practices: Case study perspectives* (pp. 486–500). University Park, IL: Barcelona Publishers.

Summer, L., & Chong, H. J. (2006). Case studies in music and imagery techniques. Published as: Music and imagery techniques with an emphasis on the Bonny Method of Guided Imagery and Music. In H. J. Chong (Ed.), *Music therapy: Techniques, methods, and models* (Korean language). Seoul, Korea: Hakjisa Publishing.

Tasney, K. (1993). Beginning the healing of incest through Guided Imagery and Music: A Jungian perspective. *Journal of the Association for Music and Imagery, 2,* 35–48.

Van Horn, P. S., Green, K. E., & Martinussen, M. (2009). Survey response rates and survey administration in counseling and clinical psychology: A meta-analysis. *Educational and Psychological Measurement* 69(3), 389–403.

Ventre, M. (2002). The individual form of the Bonny Method of Guided Imagery and Music (BMGIM). In K. E. Bruscia & D. E. Grocke (Eds.), *Guided Imagery and Music: The Bonny Method and beyond* (pp. 29–36). University Park, IL: Barcelona Publishers.

Vogt, W. P. (1999). Dictionary of statistics and methodology (2nd ed.). Thousand Oaks, CA: Sage Publications.

Walker, V. (1993). Integrating guided imagery and music with verbal psychotherapy: A case study. *Journal of the Association for Music and Imagery, 2,* 111–122.

Ward, K. (2002). A Jungian orientation to the Bonny Method. In K. E. Bruscia & D. E. Grocke (Eds.), *Guided Imagery and Music: The Bonny Method and beyond* (pp. 207–224). University Park, IL: Barcelona Publishers.

Warja, M. (1994). Sounds of music through the spiraling path of individuation: A Jungian approach to music psychotherapy. *Music Therapy Perspectives, 12*(2), 75–83.

Wesley, S. B. (2002). Guided Imagery and Music with children and adolescents. In K. E. Bruscia & D. E. Grocke (Eds.), *Guided Imagery and Music: The Bonny Method and beyond* (pp. 137–150). University Park, IL: Barcelona Publishers.

Wigle-Justice, R., & Kasayka, R. (1999). Guided Imagery and Music with cancer patients. In C. Dileo (Ed.), *Music therapy and medicine: Theoretical and clinical applications* (pp. 23–30). Silver Spring, MD: American Music Therapy Association.

Wrangsjö, B. (1994). Psychoanalysis and Guided Imagery and Music: A comparison. *Journal of the Association for Music and* Imagery, 3, 35–48.

INDEX

A

Adaptations 7, 9-10, 18, 30-2, 35, 38, 45, 47-52, 54, 65, 69, 71, 77, 83, 95
Adolescents 7, 27, 31-2, 34, 36, 39, 44-5, 52-3, 103
Ages 2, 27, 31, 34, 39, 44, 53, 58
AMI Standards 84, 89
Anxiety 5, 7, 28, 34, 38, 45-6, 58
Association for Music and Imagery (AMI) 9, 73, 81-3, 88-9, 93, 95-103
Autism 28, 96

B

Bioenergetic 57-8
BMGIM session, individual 16, 18
Bonny's Group Form 10, 17, 21
Bonny's Group GIM 70-1
Boundaries 10-11, 13, 15, 17, 21, 25, 73, 79, 82-3, 85, 89-90, 95

C

Cancer 30
Care, end-of-life 30, 32, 38
Chair, empty 68
Classical music 3, 14-15, 33-7, 39-41, 69, 71, 85-6
    selecting 36, 38
    short programs of 35, 72
    supportive 35-6, 39
Client age groups 27, 85-7
Client images 18, 44, 47, 54, 62, 86
Client transferences 61-2
Client's experience 14, 19, 28, 30, 41, 66, 69, 75, 86
Client's transferences 60-2
Components 10-23
Consciousness 3-4, 10-14, 25, 35-6, 39, 48, 50-2, 79-80, 93-5

exploration of 2, 13, 20-1, 28-9, 31, 38, 41, 46, 56, 85-6
Cotherapist 47, 61
Creation of GIM 2-7
Cultures 44

D

Dialogue 18-19, 21-3, 43, 46-8, 51, 54-5, 66, 69
DIM (Directed Imagery and Music) 65-6, 71
Directed music imaging 12-13, 18, 21, 49, 51
Directive interventions 18, 52, 68, 71-2, 74-5, 78-9, 86
Directiveness 19, 88
Dream 53-5, 68
Dream material 68
Drugs, mind-altering 2-3

E

Ego strength 29, 37, 39, 78
Existential 57-8, 80, 87-9
Existential orientation 78-9
Extemporaneous programming 33-4, 73, 81, 86

G

GAI (Guided Affective Imagery) 4
Gestalt 19, 57-8
Gestalt orientation 58
Gestalt techniques 68
GIM fellows 9, 26, 44, 73-5, 82-3, 85-9, 91
GIM programs 36, 77-8, 81, 96
    predesigned 38, 66
GIM sessions 6, 20, 26, 46-7, 49, 59, 61-2, 70-2
GIM training 9, 82, 88-90
GMI (Guided Music Imaging) 83
Goals 6, 10-11, 14-16, 20-1, 25, 37, 47, 52, 54, 66, 80, 85-7
Group co-imaging 55-6

Group format   14, 16, 53
Group forms   9-10, 17-18, 21, 57
Group GIM   14-17, 21, 23, 25, 32-3, 43, 45, 52, 54, 56, 70
   adaptations of   30, 53
Group GIM sessions   12, 14, 18, 20, 29-30, 70-2, 79
   60-minute   29
   used   31
Group go-rounds   55-6
Group Guided Imagery   100
Group reimaging   54-5
Group sessions   9, 11, 16, 18-21, 28, 30-4, 43, 45, 48, 51, 53-4, 56
   shortening of   31-2
Group work   10, 15-16, 35, 41
Groups   4-5, 16-18, 20-1, 31-3, 35, 39, 45, 49-50, 52-6, 70, 81, 87, 99
Guide   3, 5-6, 12-14, 18-21, 47-8, 50-1, 54-6, 70, 75, 81
Guiding   5, 16, 19, 21, 25, 43-56, 60, 68, 75, 78, 81, 86-7
Guiding interventions   6, 43-5
   directive   19
Guiding techniques   3, 47
   directive   68, 74

H

Healing   47, 49, 67, 70, 78, 91, 101-2
Humanistic   15, 17, 19-21,22, 23, 45, 47-8, 50, 57-9, 64, 78-9, 87-9

I

Imagery   4-6, 9-10, 35, 41, 47, 49, 54, 62, 77-80, 82-4, 86, 93, 95, 97-103
Images   4, 6, 12-13, 18, 21, 38-9, 41, 44-5, 49-52, 54-6, 64, 67, 74-5, 78, 86
Imaging, progressive group   55-6
Individual GIM sessions   6, 20, 30, 40, 71, 79
Inductions   4, 6, 20-1, 28-9, 45-9, 56, 64, 66, 68, 71, 78, 80
Institute for Consciousness and Music   94
Interventions   18, 21, 43-6, 50, 52, 54, 57, 74, 89
   nondirective   19-20, 45, 74

J

Jung 63
Jungian 22-3, 57-9, 63-4, 87
Jungian approach to GIM 63-4
Jungian archetypes in GIM therapy 101
Jungian orientations 57-8, 103
Jungian therapist 63

M

Mandalas 6, 48, 53, 74, 88
Maryland Psychiatric Research Center (MPRC) 2
MDN (Music, Drawing, and Narrative) 68-9, 72, 95
MDN sessions 69
Medical patients 30-1, 38
Modifications 10, 20-3, 25-6, 28-30, 33, 38, 43, 45-6, 48, 56-7, 59, 64-6, 73-6, 81-3, 89-90
Modified GIM 78-80, 82-4
MPD (Multiple Personality Disorder) 37, 100
Multiple Personality Disorder (MPD) 37, 100
Music, selection and use of 25, 34, 59
Music-centered approach 33, 40-1, 43, 86
Music-centered interventions 43, 45, 74-5, 86, 88
Music experience 6, 16, 18, 20, 28, 44, 60, 65-6, 68, 75, 86
Music imaging 4, 18-20, 28-32, 38, 43-53, 55-9, 66-8, 71, 73-4, 85-7
    spontaneous 12, 21, 46
Music lengths 27, 34, 78-9, 85
Music listening portions 25, 28-9, 32
Music programming 81
    spontaneous 40
Music programs 5, 26, 68-9, 78-80, 95
    50-minute 5, 20
    changed 38
    classical 11, 14, 69
    designed 5
    designing classical 5

entire 64
  predesigned 33, 36
  predesigned classical 21
  shortened 20
  shorter 29, 69
  standard predesigned 85
  taped 94
Music psychotherapy 16, 95, 103
  dynamics of 95, 98, 100, 102
Music therapists 17, 83, 96, 98
Music therapy 2, 11-12, 17, 51, 93, 95-6, 98-103
Music transference 61, 102
Myths 63

N

Nonclassical music 14, 21, 33-5, 41, 52, 71, 85
  using 85
Nontherapeutic goals 15, 17, 70-1

P

Patients 30-2, 38, 46, 48-52
Peak Experience 5-6
Physical illness 28, 30, 32, 35, 38-9, 45, 49
Physical interventions 6, 19, 43-5, 47, 74-6, 81, 86, 88
Populations 27, 34-5, 44-5, 58, 85-7
Postlude 6, 19-20, 44, 48, 50, 56-8, 68, 72, 74, 78, 87
Postlude processing 28, 30
Predesigned programs 14-15, 33-4, 36, 71, 81, 87
Prelude 6, 19-20, 28, 44-5, 48, 56-8, 65-6, 72, 74, 87
Programming 33-4, 40-1, 43, 86, 96
  music-centered 79, 81
Programs 4-5, 14, 26, 33-4, 39-41, 78, 81, 83, 99
  designing 34
  full-length 26

Programs for Guided Imagery and Music   96
Projective listening   12-13, 21, 49, 51, 69
Psychiatric   7, 28, 31-2, 35, 41, 45, 56, 85
Psychiatric clients   28, 32, 45
   individual   38
   institutionalized   28
Psychiatric clients range   32
Psychiatric patients   30, 36, 50, 99
Psychoanalysis and Guided Imagery and Music   103
Psychodynamic   17, 19-20, 22-3, 38, 57-9, 64, 87
Psychosis   44
Psychotherapy   95, 97-8, 103
PTSD (post-traumatic stress disorder)   28-9, 32, 36-7, 93

Q

Quiet Music   5

R

Re-imaging   12-13, 21-3, 66, 68, 71
Relationships   6, 60-1, 69-70, 73-6, 80, 85-8, 91, 98
Research   3, 73, 85-7, 89
Resistance   59, 61, 63, 90
Retreats   70
   spiritual   70, 72, 98

S

Session lengths   11, 20-1, 25-32, 34, 85-6
   2-hour   27
   shortened   26, 30, 32, 85
Session lengths ranging   32
Session structure   18, 74
   shorter   48
Sessions   3, 5-6, 9, 11, 15, 19-23, 25-32, 35-7, 45-7, 52-4, 56, 59-60, 68-70, 78-9, 85-6

1-hour   26
50-minute   28, 69
50-minute GIM   32
90-minute   29
drug   3, 5
individual   14, 19-21, 25, 28-9, 31-2, 34, 39, 41, 45, 48-52, 56, 64, 70-1, 85
shortened   20, 28-9, 31, 71
shortened GIM   13
shortened individual   30
standard   85
standard-length   26
used 60-minute GIM   28
Spiritual orientations   15, 57-8, 88-9, 98
Spirituality   15-16, 70-1, 94
Spontaneous imaging   4-5, 11-13, 18-19, 21, 48-9, 51, 54, 56, 66, 68, 75
Spontaneous programming   14, 21, 33, 38, 41, 89
Supportive-level work   78-9
Survey   11, 25-7, 32-3, 43-4, 47, 52, 54, 57, 65, 71, 74, 87-9, 100

T

Theoretical orientations   7, 11, 17, 19-20, 25, 38, 46, 57-64, 76, 87-8, 90
Therapeutic goals   16-17, 20, 49, 79
Therapeutic purposes   17, 21, 45, 50, 52-3, 56
Therapist   2, 6, 11-13, 18, 21, 36-8, 43-5, 47-8, 50, 54, 56, 59-62, 64-9, 74-6, 85-7
Trainers   81, 84, 89
Training   10, 73, 77, 81-4, 88-9, 93, 99
Training in Guided Imagery and Music   96
Transference   60-3, 89, 95, 100
   split   60-1
Transference objects   59, 61-2
Transpersonal   15, 22-3, 57-8, 64, 78, 80, 87-9
Transpersonal orientation   16, 19-21, 45, 47-8, 50, 59
Traumatic experience   65
Traumatized clients   29, 36, 38, 46-7

Traveler   6, 11-14, 16, 18-19, 36, 69-70

V

Variations in Length of Session and Music   26-32
Variations in Selection and Use of Music   34-41
Variations in Theoretical Orientation   58-64
Variations in Verbal Dialogue   44-56
Verbal dialogue   6, 11, 18, 25, 43-56, 73, 86-7

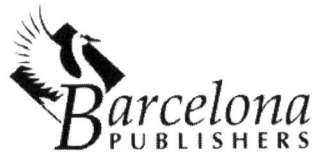

OTHER BOOKS ON
GUIDED IMAGERY AND MUSIC

Guided Imagery and Music: The Bonny Method and Beyond
(Edited by Kenneth E. Bruscia & Denise Grocke)

Music and Consciousness: The Evolution of Guided Imagery and Music
(Helen Bonny: Edited by Lisa Summer)

Music for the Imagination (10 CDs)
(Compiled by Kenneth E. Bruscia)

Case Examples of Guided Imagery and Music
(Compiled by Kenneth E. Bruscia)